MENTAL TRAINING
for
PEAK
PERFORMANCE

D1021200

ALSO BY STEVEN UNGERLEIDER, PhD

Health Resources Online: A Guide for Mental Health and Addiction Specialists, with Colette Kimball; Laura Scheerer, PhD; Glenn Meyer, PhD; and Brian Zevnik, PhD (Integrated Publishing)

Quest for Success: Legacies of Winning (WRS-Spence Press)

Beyond Strength: Psychological Profiles of Olympic Athletes, with Jacqueline M. Golding (McGraw-Hill)

Faust's Gold: Inside the East German Doping Machine (St. Martin's Press)

MENTAL TRAINING
for
PEAK
PERFORMANCE

TOP ATHLETES
REVEAL THE MIND EXERCISES
THEY USE TO EXCEL

STEVEN UNGERLEIDER, PhD

Foreword by NICK BOLLETTIERI

RODALE

In memory of my beloved friend and mentor,
Professor Milton Rosenbaum, MD

Notice

This book is intended as a reference volume only, not as a medical manual. The information given here is designed to help you make informed decisions about your health. It is not intended as a substitute for any treatment that may have been prescribed by your doctor. If you suspect that you have a medical problem, we urge you to seek competent medical help.

Mention of specific companies, organizations, or authorities in this book does not imply endorsement by the publisher, nor does mention of specific companies, organizations, or authorities imply their endorsement of this book.

Internet addresses and telephone numbers appearing in this book were accurate at the time it went to press.

© 2005 by Steven Ungerleider, PhD

All rights reserved. No part of this publication may be reproduced or transmitted in any form or by any means, electronic or mechanical, including photocopying, recording, or any other information storage and retrieval system, without the written permission of the publisher.

Printed in the United States of America
Rodale Inc. makes every effort to use acid-free ∞, recycled paper ♻.

Interior design by Drew Frantzen
Cover design by Christopher Rhoads

Library of Congress Cataloging-in-Publication Data

Ungerleider, Steven.
    Mental training for peak performance : top athletes reveal the mind exercises they use to excel / Steven Ungerleider ; foreword by Nick Bollettieri.
        p.   cm.
    Includes index.
    ISBN-13 978–1–59486–028–7 paperback
    ISBN-10 1–59486–028–9 paperback
    1. Sports—Psychological aspects.   2. Mind and body.   3. Visualization.   I. Title.
GV706.4.U555   2005
796'.01—dc22   2005014308

Distributed to the trade by Holtzbrinck Publishers

2   4   6   8   10   9   7   5   3   1   paperback

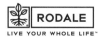

We inspire and enable people to improve their lives and the world around them
For more of our products visit **rodalestore.com** or call 800-848-4735

CONTENTS

PART THREE: SPORT-SPECIFIC MENTAL PRACTICE

FOREWORD

By Nick Bollettieri, director of Bolletieri/IMG Academies

"WHICH WOULD YOU RATHER BE: MISERABLE LIKE ARISTOTLE OR CONTENTED LIKE A PIG?"

Most of us, especially athletes, are all too familiar with the misery of Aristotle, commonly known as overthinking. Ever since the appearance of *Homo sapiens* on the planet nearly 150,000 years ago, our well-developed brains (blame it on the cerebral cortex) have enabled us to think, reason, create, and empathize—all good things—but also to worry, doubt, and obsessively self-analyze—not good things, especially if you are a tennis player serving for game, set, match, and championship at the US Open. Think of it as the "centipede effect": If the lowly centipede had to think about coordinating each of its legs to get from Point A to Point B, it would be totally immobilized—and I have worked with some athletes who were not far from that state of mind.

An immobilized brain is often the reason why the strongest or fastest or most skillful athlete will lose a competition to a competitor who, on paper at least, seems inferior. While physical skill is important, other factors determine a champion—chief among them, factors like mental conditioning, toughness, focus, and the ability to recover swiftly from a setback.

For more than 50 years, I have instructed many of the world's finest tennis players, including Andre Agassi, Boris Becker, Tommy Haas, Serena and Venus Williams, Monica Seles, Anna Kournikova, Maria Sharapova, and many others. At this level of the game, all of these players (and their opponents) have roughly similar physical and mechanical skills. Where the consistent winners outperform their opponents is in their mental abilities. They can access their physical talents "on demand." They can recover quickly, almost instantaneously, from adversity. As they say in Texas, it's not how often a cowboy falls off his horse; it's how often he gets back on.

Consider the 2004 British Open Golf Championship. The two contending players included one of the very best golfers in the world, Ernie Els, who had already won one major tournament in 2004. However, lurking in his mind, no doubt, were the inordinate number of second-place finishes he had accumulated in his career.

His opponent, Todd Hamilton, was a virtual unknown on the tour as well as to the huge spectator gallery.

As I watched Els and Hamilton, my coaching instincts told me that the winner would not be determined by who was the better hitter of the ball but by who could keep his calm and withstand the mental pressure of the moment.

And that's exactly what happened. On the 18th hole of regulation play, Hamilton got into trouble before he reached the green, and I'm sure it appeared to most viewers that Els would win the tournament. But Hamilton never changed his expression and gave no visual message that he was in trouble; in fact, to look at him, one would think that he had no worries whatsoever. His face had the perfect passivity of a world-class poker player. I'd seen that look before on the faces of champions I'd coached. Seeing it then convinced me: One mistake by Els, and Hamilton would take the match.

Then Els missed a rather easy putt, one that would have sealed his victory. The match was extended to an additional four playoff holes. And, to everyone's surprise but my own, Hamilton went on to win.

What the world witnessed that day was a match won first in Hamilton's mind and second on the course. Els had the victory in hand. Only the "tapes" he kept playing in his mind prevented him from getting to the trophy.

Displays of mental agility like Hamilton's aren't hard to find, if you're looking for them. As of this writing, Roger Federer is the number one tennis player in the world, and it appears he'll become an enduring champion. I was convinced of this not only by watching his masterful displays of technique, but by the way he never seems to buckle under adversity. During the final of the 2004 Tennis Masters Canada, held in Toronto at the new Rexall Stadium, with the players tied at 4–4, Andy Roddick was up 0–40 on Federer's serve, a point that would probably have given him the first set.

But it didn't happen. Federer was in total control of his mind and obviously believed he could still win that crucial game—and he did exactly that, going on to win the tournament.

(Of course, the importance of mental play is even more obvious when a top player falls. Federer was ousted in the first round of the 2004 Cincinnati Open after playing a sloppy match. His concentration seemed shot that day, and the results are proof enough that something was mentally off.)

Or take the Williams sisters. Few players have disrupted their opponents' mental games like Venus and Serena did a couple years ago, when they earned reputations for being unbeatable. Occasionally, their competitors—top athletes whose lives are dedicated to playing tennis—looked like lost schoolchildren on the court. The advantage this gave Serena and Venus was invaluable to their winning streaks. As a coach, you dream of your players getting such a tremendous advantage.

But as of this writing, things have changed: It now appears that Venus and Serena Williams are no longer feared on the tour. They have been injured too often and beaten too often (sometimes lopsidedly as in the 2004 Wimbledon final when Maria Sharapova easily defeated Serena in two short sets). Can the Williams sisters come back? Of course they can—they're both great champions—but the edge (and, therefore, the mental advantage) of being thought of as invincible may never return. To get there, it will take some tough mental work by Venus and Serena themselves.

As Dr. Ungerleider will teach us in this book, mental conditioning, focus, and toughness are learnable skills and techniques that all world-class athletes employ—and you can, too. His work is an invaluable guide to the fascinating, largely unmapped, territory of the mind. For athletes (or anyone) looking for peak performance in their lives, this task is an essential road map.

ACKNOWLEDGMENTS

I want to thank my buddies at Rodale, including Jeremy Katz, Daniel Listwa, Chris Krogermeier, Rose Panetta, and the creative team. And a very special thanks to Courtney Conroy, my editor at Rodale.

Many thanks to Halle Reese, Dr. Randa Ryan and her colleagues at UT, and Adam Jonas, my terrific research assistant. Also thanks to Nick Bollettieri, Roger Staubach, Steve Jones, and Jerry Jones of the Dallas Cowboys organization and to Jeremy Halbraich, Michael Levin, and Stu Perlmeter. And words of gratitude to Steve Baum, David Ulich, Bill Mason, and Janice Silvernail of Justice for Athletes. Many kudos to my staff at Integrated Research, my wonderful and trusted assistant, Jan Bartunek; Colette Kimball, MPH; Colie Mason; IT guru Jerry Nordahl; and Wil Scott. And thanks to Sharon.

More thanks to US Senator Ben Nighthorse Campbell, my attorney and advisor Hans David Ulich of Sheppard Mullin, and to all of the agents and lawyers and federations who assisted me with access to athlete interviews. To my mentors, J. Thomas Ungerleider, MD, and Professor Martin Acker— I offer appreciation for many years of support. Special thanks to IMG for their wonderful assistance. Additional thanks to friend and support team, MLBB and Richard W. Pound and his superb team at WADA. And a special thanks to the Mayhew family.

And to my girls, Shoshana (pc/pbk) and Ariel (tb), thanks for being my daughters and my best friends!

INTRODUCTION

Welcome to the fully revised and updated *Mental Training for Peak Performance*! Since 1996, when this book was first published, I've spent a great amount of time writing and commentating on the history of steroid use in sports, as documented in my last book, *Faust's Gold*. Now, in this fully revised and updated version of *Mental Training for Peak Performance*, I happily return to my roots—understanding how and why athletes use mental rehearsal in preparing for their events. For that matter, how do any of us—lawyers, doctors, chefs, corporate execs, students—use mental practice techniques? And do they work? Through my study of the phenomenon of mental training with my colleague, Jacqueline Golding, PhD, of the University of California, San Francisco, we found that the answer is yes! We surveyed 1,200 Olympians in the mid-1980s. Our results, published in *Beyond Strength: Psychological Profiles of Olympic Athletes* (McGraw-Hill, 1990), were quite exciting. Mental practice, including mental, auditory, and kinesthetic imagery, all work. And, when implemented properly and with some guidance, they can lead to astonishing success.

In the first part of this revised edition, you will find a clear explanation of the techniques and why athletes use them. You will learn that athletes who use mental training techniques are more relaxed, better prepared, and often more successful. In the second part, you will learn how to use the mental training and rehearsal techniques yourself. Each technique is clearly explained, both in theory and application.

The third part will offer insights and examples from top athletes of many disciplines, including an all-new chapter on mental training for pentathletes. This section will include insights into how elite competitors use mental practice to optimize their performances. You'll find tips on how you can incorporate these techniques into your training to enhance your skills. You'll find ways to improve your performance in any sport, with recommendations and examples from some of the world's most prominent athletes. In these pages, I will discuss motivation, commitment to training, cross-training, pain thresholds, fatigue, and overtraining. These recommendations apply to the developmental athlete, the high school competitor, the you-and-me–type recreational athlete, and the elite competitor.

I have also added a list, updated as of 2005, of athletic federations, contact info, and Web sites for more information. Also, for those athletes who want to understand the problems and serious health consequences surrounding nutritional supplements, drugs, and other performance-enhancement issues, I have also included Web sites and phone contacts.

From this material, I hope you will continue to build your own mental practice program and strengthen your performance in whichever sport you choose. The information in these pages will help you boost your confidence, enhance your self-esteem, and increase your athletic competence—all the ingredients you need to reach your potential peak performance.

PART ONE

INTRODUCTION TO MENTAL TRAINING

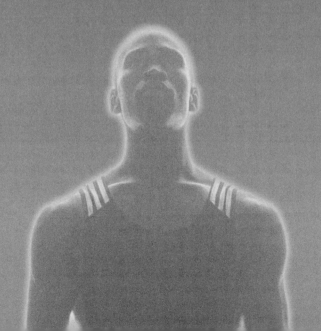

CHAPTER 1

What Mental Training Can Do for You

One of the great moments in Olympic competition was during the final event at the 1992 Barcelona Games. Trent Dimas, a member of the US Men's Olympic Gymnastics Team, prepared to mount the horizontal bar for the last event before closing ceremonies. His bar routine was flawless, with stunning form and absolute body control on all his optional tricks. Even more spectacular were his release moves: letting go of the high bar in midair and cruising through space with grace and elegance. In anticipation of a perfect landing, he started smiling even before he dismounted from the apparatus, planting both feet firmly on the ground. The judges rewarded him with a perfect 10; to have done otherwise would have been a great injustice.

Watching him again on the television replay in the days following the Games was, to some degree, even more exciting. As the camera zoomed in on Dimas just seconds before he began his journey of swings, releases, and awesome catches on the bar, the slow-motion television replay captured a moment of quiet solitude, a moment of reflection, a moment of mental preparation. Dimas closed his eyes and just waited patiently for his routine to flash before his mental "imagery disk," replaying the visuals one more time so his actual event would be in sync with what his mind and body were feeling.

Trent Dimas, en route to winning his gold medal, was calling on his mental practice training to help ensure a flawless performance.

THE WINNING DIFFERENCE

Before the 1988 Olympic Games in Seoul, social psychologist Jacqueline Golding, PhD, and I surveyed 1,200 track and field athletes who qualified for the Olympic Trials. We specifically compared athletes who qualified for the Olympic Games with those who nearly qualified but missed. We found that these two groups of athletes had a lot in common. You could say they all had "the right stuff." They were training hard, eating right, getting plenty of sleep, avoiding alcohol and other intoxicants, and using their brains as well as their brawn to compete. They were nearly identical in every respect except for one thing.

Those athletes who actually made the team and competed in the Olympics were doing more mental practice in the final stages of preparation than their less-successful colleagues. The athletes who actually qualified for the Olympics were doing final "mental tune-ups" and getting ready for the competitive challenge of their lives: the Olympic Games. We learned from our studies with Olympians that mental preparation and the timing of mental preparation are the keys to who succeeds.

This type of mental practice is exactly what gymnast Trent Dimas was doing just before his flawless gold-medal performance. I asked Dimas's coach, Ed Burch of Gold Cup Gymnastics in Albuquerque, New Mexico, about this performance ritual. Burch explained that all his athletes, including two-time Olympian Lance Ringnald, practiced mental rehearsal, using the visualization strategies appropriate for their particular events.

"It is standard procedure for all my gymnasts, including Trent," said Burch. "I told Trent that he had to spend the night before finals in his room in the Olympic Village mentally rehearsing his routine. I retired early that night as well, didn't party like the rest of the gang, and spent a few hours mentally preparing for his event. So when you speak about mental practice or the magic of visualization, it goes both ways. Coaches who know their athletes work together in physical training and in mental preparation as well."

NOW EVERYONE DOES IT

Mental training is now an accepted part of many training programs. I think that we have entered an era where athletes can honestly say, "I won because I trained hard both physically and psychologically."

Mark Plaatjes, gold-medal winner in the Men's Marathon at the 1993 Track and Field World Championship in Stuttgart, Germany, attributes much of his success to being ready. "I was so mentally prepared, it was scary," he says. "I even started to worry that things were too perfect. I had received some information and pictures on the contours and flow of the marathon course prior to arriving in Germany. When I got to Stuttgart, I felt completely comfortable and absolutely familiar with the course. There's no doubt that I was the most motivated runner in my marathon race, but I was also the most prepared."

When I first got involved in sport psychology, I remember traveling to California State University, Hayward, to participate in a mental tune-up session with competitive ice skaters under the tutelage of Betty Wenz, PhD. I remember lying on the rather cold and uncomfortable locker room floor with 25 skaters as Dr. Wenz took us through a series of visual images to assist the skaters with their training techniques. I wonder how many of those gifted kids took those mental practice gems to the ice.

By the time Dr. Golding and I began our studies in the 1980s, mental practice was more common. Nearly all of the Olympians we surveyed going into the 1988 Seoul Games had heard of imagery, visualization, or mental practice, and most of them understood the concept. An amazing 83 percent—524 athletes of 633 who responded to our survey—practiced some form of it. These results told me that we were no longer living in the dark ages as far as imagery and visualization were concerned.

Margaret Groos, 1988 Olympic marathoner and winner of the US Trials, told me after her fabulous race: "I know that my mental preparation for the marathon helped me in my training. Usually, I imagined certain points in the race—catching someone, pulling away from another, or the finish of the race. If you haven't done your mental homework in training, then you don't have anything to fall back on when you race."

Mental homework rings true for me in almost anything I do, including writing this book. If I'm not prepared with a set of images that lay out conceptual frameworks for my chapters, I can spend all day just staring at my

(continued on page 8)

WHY MENTAL PRACTICE WORKS

There are some 100 research studies documenting the effects of mental practice and imagery on athletic performance. Many sport scientists have spent most of their careers trying to understand this delicate relationship. Debra Feltz, PhD, and Dan Landers, PhD, well-known researchers in sport psychology, have studied how and when mental practice best improves performance.

When I first wrote this book, I highlighted two possible explanations behind why mental practice and, more specifically, imagery work: the symbolic learning theory and the psychoneuromuscular theory. Since then, experts have focused on an additional two reasons, known as the bio-informational theory and the dual coding theory.

Here is what we know about all four.

1. **Symbolic learning theory.** Imagery may be part of a coding system that actually helps athletes understand movement. The theory says that every move we make in life is first coded like a blueprint in our minds and in our nervous systems, so that if we mentally rehearse an athletic event, we are actually blueprinting each move, making the gestures symbolic and making them more familiar to our body chemistry. By doing lots of mental practice, we are setting the stage for movement to become quite automatic and easy to recall.

For example, if Andy Roddick and Jennifer Capriati want to improve their backhand crosscourt shots, they might break out each component of the task by mentally rehearsing each sequence of the tennis shot. In this way they would encode each movement of their hands, wrists, forearms, and elbows, creating a blueprint for the entire backhand tennis swing. This familiarity would enhance their shots and make them relaxed, strong, and incredibly accurate. Dramatic improvements in basketball free-throw shooting are credited to the symbolic learning theory.

2. **Psychoneuromuscular theory.** Mental practice works because even when we sit quietly in our armchairs, we are actually producing very small muscle contractions similar to those involved in our particular sport.

Let's examine this theory, using the mind of Olympic diving champion Greg Louganis as an example. Theoretically, when Louganis concentrates on his sport, his mind shoots mental "faxes" and other electronic impulses to his muscles and tendons, reminding them how to leap from the springboard, prepare to tuck, rotate for several spins, and then unravel the body for a perfect no-splash entry into the pool. These messages travel at lightning speed and cause the muscles to fire at appropriate sequences so they can perform the correct sporting movement. In essence, they allow Louganis's muscles to practice, even when his body is at rest.

This theory has been tested quite frequently by simply having athletes mentally rehearse images and then measuring the electrical activity (with an electromyograph, or EMG) in their arms and legs. In one experiment, a psychologist in Colorado measured the electrical activity of a downhill ski racer while the skier sat quietly imaging the race course. The printout of the racer's leg muscle contractions and firings corresponded exactly to the terrain of the hilly and challenging ski course. If we mentally rehearse our sports often and with great intensity, we strengthen and condition the muscle firings and neuromuscular "phone lines" so that the messages get there more efficiently and with greater clarity.

3. **Bio-informational theory.** This third theory, first brought to light by doctors trying to explain the connection between imagery and anxiety disorders, states that if we imagine how we might respond to a certain event, we can better prepare for it.

For instance, if Tiger Woods had a problem with anxiety and nerves while putting, it would be helpful for him to go home and imagine making putts while being anxious and nervous. That way, when he hit the links, he would already be used to the anxiety and actually begin to feel (almost paradoxically) comfortable when the anxiety hit. This would ultimately allow the anxiety to disappear and let him play better.

(continued)

WHY MENTAL PRACTICE WORKS (*cont.*)

4. **Dual coding theory.** This theory suggests that athletes receive information by two independent channels or encoding systems, the verbal channel and the motor channel. Simply stated, this means that new skills are better learned if they are both explained to an athlete and then actualized through physical practice. The link between the two channels is known as the action-language bridge.

The bridge is the key to athletic learning and success here: It makes it possible for athletes to describe an action, generate another action, and act on verbal cues. For example, if Woods were to go back to Stanford, his alma mater, to give a lecture on how he swings, he might first talk players through his mechanics (the verbal part) and then walk players through practicing his swing (the motor part) while describing it again. The players would thus be learning on two different levels and bridging between them through Woods's instruction.

word processor, accomplishing little. You'll find the same to be true for you in most of your activities, whether you're doing routine daily tasks or training to reach your athletic goals.

PRESSING YOUR SENSES INTO SERVICE

Mental practice and imagery are not exactly the same, but they are very similar. Mental practice simply means repeating a task in your mind, without any movement from your body. Imagery, however, is a very specific and very focused type of mental practice. Imagery can be described as an exercise that uses all of the senses to create an experience in the mind.

Visualization is just one part of this imagery experience. We can also feel, smell, taste, hear, and touch in our imagery experience. Watching a videotape of diver Julie Ogenhouse at the 1992 Barcelona Summer Olympics offers a wonderful example of the different senses that you might experience in imagery practice.

As Ogenhouse prepares to dive, she uses her eyes to note the distance of the springboard from the water; she uses her sense of speed and motion to decide how best to rotate on the 3½ front somersault with a 1½ twist; she hears the sound of the board as it rebounds from her thrust; she feels the simple, yet perfect, splash of the water against her body on entry; she smells the chlorine from the pool water; then she receives the energy of the crowd when the dive is complete.

Utilizing all the senses, an athlete like Ogenhouse also focuses on the importance of emotions. Competitive athletes use imagery to help control anxiety, anger, or pain. Athletes who learn these skills recreate emotions in their minds to enhance the quality of their performances. When imagery is used effectively, the learning process becomes exciting and opens up a whole realm of human potential.

Laura Wilkinson is an extreme example of someone tapping into the power of imagery. Going into the 2000 Sydney Olympics, dive champion Wilkinson broke her leg and was in a cast for months. She could not dive—physically, that is. But by working with a supportive coach and using imagery practice, Wilkinson was able to stay focused. Several times each day, she'd climb the 10-meter platform and "walk" through the motions of her complex high dives, mentally taking snapshots of each element. When the cast came off just before the Sydney games, she got up on the 10-meter platform and did some very elegant dives. Wilkinson's practice was so good, she lost very little training time and went on to win the gold in Sydney.

We all know friends who go out and attempt to imitate the tennis serve of Pete Sampras or emulate the great reflexes of Andre Agassi—and they might do quite well. After watching the phenomenal skills of Steve Kerr in the NBA finals, you may be inspired to go out and shoot three-pointers, surprising yourself by sinking one after another. So is there a relationship between watching the very best and then imitating that outstanding athletic feat?

The answer is yes.

Imagery becomes a dynamic element in the learning process. Athletes imitate the actions of others, because their minds "take a picture" of the activity, and they use it as a model for their performances. Anyone can model his physical performance using this kind of mental "filming." Imagery is based on memory, and we experience it internally by reconstructing external events in our minds. As the programmer of our own imagery tapes, we are able to build an image from whatever pieces of memory we choose.

Len Spencer, a tennis pro and my daughter's talented coach, explained to me many years ago that unpleasant events can directly affect performance. He noted that if our memories are laced with traumatic or frustrating moments on the court or off-court pressure from an overbearing parent, we tend to lock "trauma images" into our muscle memory and not perform well. He used to call to me from the sidelines, "Steven, get your computer and your office work out of the picture, relax your grip, get your feet in motion, and enjoy the game." I can still hear his voice barking those commands.

OUT OF THE DARK AGES

In the past several decades, dramatic changes have occurred in the way athletes prepare, train, and compete at all levels of sport. As coaches have turned to a more mind-body approach to training, athletes have responded with improved performances and greater longevity in their sports. It is no secret that great athletes such as tennis stars Pete Sampras, Andre Agassi, and Martina Navratilova; basketball legend Michael Jordan; and pitchers Randy Johnson and Roger Clemens have stayed fit longer, kept their bodies healthier, and remained competitive well beyond their supposed peak performance years. Martina Navratilova personified the trend when she competed in doubles at the US Open at age 48, making it to the semifinal round.

These athletes are going years beyond their performance window of opportunity by using alternative strategies that include mental practice and visualization. Their training programs address their complete needs, from nutrition to stress management to creative mental preparation and performance strategies. These mental training strategies enhance performance while discouraging physical overtraining—which may lead to injury and burnout.

According to some sports medicine specialists from the former Eastern bloc nations, mental practice strategies have been a regular part of training elite-level athletes since the 1960s. Several experts note that Romania and several other Eastern European countries initially train their coaches in mental preparation strategies, and in turn, the coaches train their athletes. This style of teaching and training differs dramatically from our Western model. In the United States, for example, sport psychologists work with athletes first (and sometimes exclusively) and then hope that coaches will participate in mental preparation training as the athletes improve their performances.

While it may be preferable to have coaches help with the mental training process, it apparently isn't essential. In the survey that Dr. Golding and I conducted, we found that many athletes who trained without coaches had designed innovative mental practice strategies on their own and incorporated them into their daily training.

You don't have to have a coach to lead you to the well. The visualization spring is always full of water and is available to anyone who takes a drink. No doubt certain coaches, such as gymnastics coach Burch—who does visualization work with his athletes—inspire a certain synergistic relationship with athletes who are willing to work hard and prepare diligently for their sports.

Finally, athletes at any level—not just elite athletes—can benefit from mental training. Even after exhaustive research with hundreds of athletes, I do not need to go very far to see results. My daughters (who are now young women well into their academic and athletic careers) vouch for mental practice. My younger daughter, Ariel, a former gymnast and now a Division I collegiate cheerleader and stunter, told me, "Dad, I often see myself doing the perfect round-off, back handspring into a full; it's so clear, and I can feel the mat beneath my hands—and I'm just lying in my bed getting ready for sleep."

CHAPTER 2

Mental Training Secrets
of Competitive Athletes

Maria Mutola, the four-time Olympian and 800-meter Olympic and World Championship gold medalist, has told me, "Just before I get ready to race, especially the big ones, I will do some relaxation, listen to music, a bit of mental tune-up, and some prayers." She explained to me over lunch that each has its place in the mental training sequence. "If I don't prepare with each element (relaxation, the music, mental tune-up, and prayer), I will know immediately that I'm not fully prepared. I have to have each piece in the proper sequence and with a full commitment before I race, or my emotional balance will be off."

Mutola did a good piece of mental prep in September 2003 at the IAAF Grand Slam in Brussels when she won gold—again—and took home $1 million in prize money, the largest sum ever paid to a female track athlete in history.

All of us would love to have the athletic and mental skills of Mutola and other great athletes. All of us would love to transform negative images into positive ones; replace old visual cues with new, performance-enhanced ones; and use our dreams to map interventions for winning events. These are the ingredients that work for Olympic athletes and recreational athletes as well.

HOW TOP ATHLETES SEE IMAGES

Have you ever played tennis with a friend and sensed that you weren't all there? You might have felt as if you were watching yourself from the sidelines—not focusing on your game, but actually being a spectator. I asked the Olympians whom I surveyed with Jacqueline Golding, PhD, if they use imagery to see themselves run through a skill. (Most did.) Then I asked, "If so, do you see yourself from the outside (as if watching a video screen), or do you experience the skill from the inside (as if you are actually inside yourself performing)?"

About a third of these Olympians saw themselves from both inside *and* outside. About ⅓ observed from within, or an inside view, and a similar number observed from outside, or a video view. What does all this mean, and is it relevant to a competitive strategy?

Carmen Troncoso, a 5000-meter Olympian, explained to me that imagery perspective comes in different forms, shapes, and doses. "I just picture myself (internally) in the race and try to think of all the possible things (externally) that can go wrong, and then shift that to all the things I want to go right. It's a lot easier to do imagery once you know who is out there competing against you and what times they run. And then I just review the race over and over and avoid all the negative images that come to mind, and just focus on a great mental race."

Clarity of images is also important. Mac Wilkins, gold-medal winner in the discus throw in the 1976 Montreal Games, commented: "Between Montreal, Los Angeles, and Seoul, the difference was clarity of my focus— clarity of my vision or even my ability to visualize what my target was and how to get there. In 1976 it was crystal clear . . . that clarity was not so sharp, however, in Los Angeles . . . and I knew it, and it bothered me."

For some reason younger athletes had clearer images when they rehearsed the various elements of their sports. Here is where it gets interesting. The images that the US Olympians recalled tended to be associated with strong emotions, with half the athletes choosing a very strong emotion tied to the imagery process. When javelin throwers prepare their approach for the javelin throw, for example, there is a sense of power and tension. This emotion "pumps up" the individual so that he can prepare the mind and body to throw the javelin. Only 1 in 10 of the athletes said their images did not conjure up strong emotions.

(continued on page 16)

WHO USES MENTAL PRACTICE?

In the 1980s, social psychologist Jacqueline Golding, PhD, and I began in-depth studies of athletes. First, we studied masters track and field athletes who had competed in the 1984 and 1987 US Championships. In 1987, we initiated our survey of 1,200 Olympic track and field athletes, the largest one ever conducted in the United States. These athletes, qualifiers for the Olympic Trials in 43 track and field events, were sent 16-page, 240-item questionnaires that covered physical and mental training strategies, injuries, mood, motivation, and social support. We surveyed them in April 1988 before the trials and again in November 1988 after the Games; 633 athletes responded to the initial survey and 450 responded to the follow-up survey.

We found that almost all athletes had heard of imagery, visualization, or mental practice and understood the concept, and 83 percent reported practicing some form of it. Equal numbers of men and women reported using mental practice techniques, regardless of whether or not they had a coach.

We also found that older and better-educated athletes tended to use mental practice. Eighty-eight percent of college graduates used mental training, as did 86 percent of those with graduate degrees and 57 percent of those with a high school education or less. It's possible that older may mean wiser and that more widely read individuals are more likely to discover mental training—or college coaches may steer athletes to mental training.

When did athletes use mental practice? Ninety-nine percent said they practiced before competition in bed before sleep, right before race day or a gradual buildup to the biggest event in their lives. Almost a third practiced during the event, and one in five practiced afterward.

Here's the breakdown on how often these elite athletes used mental practice.

- Once a week or less: about one in three

- Twice a week: one in five

- Three to six times a week: about one in three

- More than seven times a week: one in 10

We also found that those who trained the longest hours reported more mental training. The extra hours of training, however, could be mental training rather than physical. And, of course, the more committed athletes are more likely to train more hours, both physically and mentally, and to seek out ways to enhance their performances—such as mental practice.

Athletes who had visited a sports medicine specialist were more likely to use mental practice than athletes who had not. I found this most puzzling. After further thought and investigation, I came up with a potential explanation. A visit to a sports physician suggests an athletic injury, and some injured athletes use mental practice because they can't practice physically. It is also possible that athletes who seek out this kind of specialist for medical treatment are the same ones who seek out special cognitive techniques, both representing commitment to state-of-the-art training.

It really does work!!

More reports coming from my colleagues around the world note that imagery and visualization skills are really being used. We knew they worked, but now we have convinced the coaches and athletes. My colleague, Jean Williams, PhD, noted in her outstanding book, *Applied Sport Psychology,* that 99 percent of the 235 Canadian Olympians who went to the 1984 Los Angeles Olympics used imagery. Forty elite gymnasts reported extensive use of imagery skill for preparation, and in 1988 some 86 percent of our US consultants used mental training strategies with our US Olympians going into the Seoul games. We know from Barcelona (1992), Atlanta (1996), Nagano (1998), Sydney (2000), Salt Lake City (2002), and Athens (2004)—I attended all of those great competition venues—that we had more psychologists working with more athletes than ever before. I would say that we are finally catching up to the Eastern bloc countries on the mental training and visualization skill learning curve.

Grigori Raiport, MD, past president of the Russian Success Method Training Center, has suggested that Russian athletes learned long ago that while the human body has its natural limits, the mind's potential is unlimited. He noted in an issue of the *Sport Psychologist* journal: "The strategic goal of Soviet sport psychology . . . is to elicit peak performance from athletes. To that end, Russians analyzed the nature of athletic inspiration and discovered that it consists of three components: physical, emotional, and mental thoughts. The Russian method is designed to train athletes to reproduce those thoughts and feelings at will, using autoconditioning. This technique helps athletes choose their optimal mood for a competition, be it joy, happiness, or anger. Even such a negative emotion as sorrow can be used constructively."

Dr. Raiport noted that any strong emotion possesses energy, and therefore, coaches might even transform the negative energy of grief into a constructive force. Take, for instance, the extraordinary gold medal performance of pentathlon Olympian, Anita Allen. Days before her competition in August 2003 at the Dominican Republic Pan Am Games, Allen lost her best friend and classmate in the Iraq war. She turned her grief into a very focused competitive win and a huge emotional release. (More about Anita and her mental toughness in the chapter on pentathlon and cross-training.)

Through my studies of both elite competitors and field athletes, I've found that elite competitors perceived controlling the picture of athletic images as slightly easier than controlling the feeling of their images. Field athletes perceived control of the picture as more difficult. I concluded that field athletes, besides possessing other qualities relating to mental practice, use their sense of "feel" more than other sensations, such as sound or sight, in approaching these strategies. For field athletes, apparently, mental practice is more important in the outcome than in some other competitions.

An athlete's control of his imagery process may open some doors to learning more about how he improves his skill level in any sport. Imagery control, however, can have both positive and negative consequences. Pole vaulter Earl Bell, a four-time member of the Olympic Team (1976 through 1988) and bronze medalist in the 1984 Los Angeles Olympics, explained to me: "Mental imagery control requires more than just a quiet place for concentration. The visuals and images that go along with the mental practice happen at an involuntary level—so that maybe you don't have complete control over yourself. Sometimes images happen best when you're not in control of everything."

BENEFITS IN THE FIELD

In our study, we found that field athletes visualized more frequently than anyone else. Here are some of our findings.

- Field athletes (pole vaulters, discus throwers, high jumpers, and such) were more likely to use mental practice and had stronger physical sensations associated with imagery than track competitors (sprinters, for example).

- 80 percent of Olympic field athletes visualized during competition, while only 50 percent of non-Olympians did.

- 50 percent of female Olympic field athletes visualized after competition, while 20 percent of female non-Olympians did.

It's possible that throwers, jumpers, vaulters, and other field competitors use mental practice more frequently than those in other events because field events have a large visual component. In fact, many field athletes have commented that it is easier to do imagery and imagery correction when you can stop, visualize your performance, and then set or correct the images before proceeding. At the 1984 Games in Los Angeles, two-time Olympian Dwight Stones was renowned for locking in his images or shaking his head when he didn't lock in prior to his approach on the high jump.

Track and field competitors may need to factor in environmental concerns such as weather, crowds, noise level, and artificial surfaces in order to access a complete picture of their success.

Marathoners we studied were less likely than track athletes to use mental practice before their events. Marathoners have more difficulty with the visual component and therefore visualize less frequently, possibly because of fatigue and other distractions during a long race. Marathon competitors also may be focusing on survival and monitoring pain as opposed to setting up imagery strategies. As 1988 Olympic marathoner Nancy Ditz put it, "Hot weather is always difficult for me. So visualizing running in hot, humid conditions is an important part of my training. I just visualize it being hot—and not feeling warm." Her technique is to imagine the absolute worst-case scenario and then respond positively to it.

These are the gems, the secrets, and the training guidelines that we need to articulate to our children and to team and individual competitors in every aspect of sport preparation. As gifted Olympic marathoner Margaret Groos reminded me, "I know instantly if it's going to be my race or not. I feel effortless—a floating sensation. I feel like the race is taking care of itself. I have that feeling every once in a while in workouts, too. . . . It's just this psychological thing where I feel very focused."

PART TWO

MENTAL TRAINING
TECHNIQUES THAT WORK

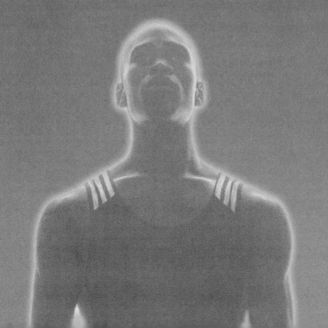

CHAPTER 3

Build Confidence with Affirmations and Self-Talk

Bruce Jenner used to interpret increased heartbeat, muscle tremor, rapid breathing, increased sweating, and a need to urinate just before the decathlon as a sign that he was nervous, excessively aroused, and wasn't going to do well. These thoughts inevitably led to a self-fulfilling prophecy. Over time, he reframed those feelings and thoughts and told himself that he was ready, prepared both physically and psychologically, and that those symptoms were a sign of readiness and positive signals to compete. The result? An Olympic gold in the decathlon in 1976. I saw him compete in the Olympic trials a few months before, and he definitely shifted his focus between the trials and his tremendous performance in Montreal.

My friend and colleague, the late Dorothy Harris, PhD, who was a professor of sport psychology at Pennsylvania State University in University Park, used to say, "The only difference between the best performance and the worst performance is the variation in our self-talk and the self-thoughts and attitudes we carry around with us." Dr. Harris was not only speaking of sport but also life in general. During her career, she wrote many articles and books and spoke about the relationship of self-talk to attitudes and behavior—right up until a few days before her death from pancreatic cancer. After her initial cancer diagnosis, she challenged her doctors by declaring that she would outlive their medical predictions by more than a year. For years she had practiced imagery, visualization, and positive affirmation strategies, and she believed this would improve her health. She won the bet and outlived the doctors' prognosis by 2 years!

THE POWER OF PAST EVENTS

Dr. Harris and others have written extensively about the fact that our awareness in sporting events goes way beyond what is happening at the moment when we compete. Our awareness level during a tennis match, for example, is triggered by earlier events and memories of previous matches. We often find ourselves searching the unconscious for memories of the past, when we were in similar situations. Most of us go back to those situations in our minds and reflect on how that previous match affected us and our performance.

We then take an inventory of that previous competitive situation and decide how we are going to play this match based on the pleasant or unpleasant thoughts that surrounded that previous event. If we had unpleasant experiences in the past, negative thoughts might seep into our minds, affecting our muscle control and overall self-image of how we might play the game today. If we had prior pleasant athletic experiences, the feelings of competence, usefulness, and high self-esteem might reemerge at the appropriate moments. These emotions and experiences have a way of becoming self-fulfilling prophecies that either work to our advantage or disadvantage.

When we talk about building confidence with affirmations and self-talk, it is important to look at the link between self-confidence and success. Certain athletes have been able to build on their confidence through years of positive thinking and reminding themselves of positive outcomes brought about by positive affirmations. These are athletes who do not give up, even though they may be four games behind in a tennis match or a quarter-mile behind in a marathon.

Tennis great Pete Sampras, who retired in August 2003 after a stunning career, is one who uses positive affirmations and self-talk to remind himself that he can conquer an opponent even if he is behind and not playing well. He will often remind himself that he has been on this court before, played the same opponent, and now needs to shift gears with some positive self-talk reminders that "everything is okay." Kenny Moore, two-time Olympic marathoner, never gave up in the grueling 26.2-mile race, even though he often experienced pain and fatigue in the last 4 to 5 miles. He told me over lunch recently, "I often reminded myself of growing up in Oregon and training on those cold, wet nights. It was tough, and I know I can work through this experience as well."

BOOSTING BELIEF IN YOUR ABILITY

Most of us don't even realize that we spend a good deal of time talking to ourselves. We are unaware of this internal dialogue; we just know that we are feeling some discomfort. Nevertheless, thoughts directly affect feelings and, ultimately, athletic movement and activity. Negative thoughts lead to negative feelings, low self-esteem, and poor performance. How can we turn these thoughts around to create positive emotions, peak performance, and a belief that we are consistent winners?

Confident athletes such as Moore and Sampras think positively, use self-talk to build on their confidence, and believe in affirmations. They focus on mastering their sports and not on worrying about poor performance or negative consequences of failure. Building on previous success and not dwelling on failure or poor performance fosters a positive self-image, confidence, and personal belief for the "can-do" athlete. In talking to a gaggle of top Olympic coaches (for instance, Russ Hellickson, head wrestling coach at Ohio State University in Columbus and two-time Olympic silver medalist), I learned that effective coaching begins by building an individual inventory of positive outcomes.

So when a coach works with a top-ranked tennis player like Sampras, the coach needs to take stock of the physical and emotional strengths of a given performance, then remind the player that he has the skills to do better after a particular match. The coach is in a unique position to observe court presence, shot selection, and footwork and reiterate performance objectives and goals so that the player can enhance his sense of worth and self-confidence. This initiates and reinforces the player's feeling of power and internal control, which builds the athlete's confidence in his tennis performance.

To be able to build confidence with affirmations, athletes have to genuinely believe in themselves. My colleague, sport psychologist Jim Loehr, PhD, founding director of sport sciences for the United States Tennis

Association and cofounder of LGE Sport Science Training Center in Orlando, Florida, has worked with some of the top tennis players in the world. These players have wonderful physiological gifts. They hit hard with great precision and their reflexes are swift, but many lack basic confidence and have very low self-images. The key, says Dr. Loehr, is to identify when and where their self-concept breaks down and try to intervene with positive self-talk and affirmations that foster strength, grace, and consistency in their tennis strokes. Positive intentions can result in positive outcomes.

Dr. Loehr suggests that we have to get to "basic confidence and early images of success," and other sport psychologists express the same sentiments. For some athletes, this might mean going back and exploring childhood concerns, fear of failure, embarrassment, humiliation among friends and family, and childhood trauma. This base of understanding builds consistently, right up to and during competition.

Mel Rosen, 1992 Olympic track and field coach and former track and field coach at Auburn University in Alabama, used to approach one of his student athletes, a three-time Olympic sprint champion, with a keen and sensitive eye to building last-minute confidence and self-image. "I would see Harvey Glance with his head down before the Olympic Trials and know that he wasn't emotionally prepared to race. I would remind him of his other big races, remind him of his need for positive self-talk and positive images when he set up in the blocks. Most of all, I would tell Harvey to keep his head up and remind him that he was the best in the business and that he could get the job done."

Glance, now head coach at the University of Alabama, uses a similar but more elaborate formula to build confidence levels. He writes notes to his athletes congratulating them on their workouts and reminding them to stay positive and refreshed when they train. He reminds them to keep a healthy and positive attitude in their daily workouts so that they can bring these images and affirmations to each race.

PERSONAL PEP TALKS

What does self-talk mean, and how does it affect athletic performance? The frequency and content of thoughts vary from individual to individual and situation to situation. Anytime you think about something, you are "talking to yourself," which is a type of self-talk.

Affirmations, on the other hand, are a very specific and individualized type of self-talk. For instance, if I say to myself before shooting white-water rapids, "Steven, stay focused," that's self-talk. Affirmations, however, would be more specific to me. I might say to myself, "I know I'm really good at doing this. I know my emotional state. I'm very positive."

Self-talk and self-affirmation become great emotional strengths when they enhance self-esteem and self-worth. It works to great advantage when this self-improvement leads to a terrific performance.

Here's how self-talk works. Pete Sampras, whom I mentioned earlier, tended to let anger trap him as a child, and he allowed it to lead to negative tension on the court. To combat this tendency, Sampras says positive things to himself, such as, "I need to get out of this mind-set," "I need to let go of that last point and stay focused on the present," and "I need to stay focused on the present and prepare for the next point." When Sampras does that, he stays fresher, he is less easily distracted, and his mind is more receptive to being able to focus on the game.

Such positive talk and affirmation may help an athlete stay in the present, completely focused on the task at hand. These mental skills may allow an athlete to perform at peak output, while blocking out images or thoughts from previous unsuccessful events. Ideally, the ultimate goal of affirmation and self-talk skill development may be to help the athlete's actions become automatic, yet intuitive. Allowing the athlete to feel and sense his way through a competition is the path to a peak performance. Most athletes at any level of sport rarely go through a competitive event without some degree of thought or feeling. Therefore, it's best to try and make those thoughts and feelings positive ones.

It is important for coaches to teach competitors how to recognize and control those thoughts. It's not the thinking itself that leads to poor performance, but rather, misguided or inappropriate thinking. These are concepts that noted sport psychologist Jean Williams, PhD, has written about and discussed extensively in her work with college and Olympic athletes. She recommends that athletes learn positive self-talk and affirmations so that they can correct bad habits, prepare for performance, focus attention, build confidence and competence, and create a positive constructive mood.

The ultimate goal of teaching self-talk and positive affirmations is to have the athlete achieve a sense of mastery—a proficiency that becomes automatic. This takes time, however, and you have to begin with the fundamentals. A coach or parent might want to suggest a cue word—a simple reminder that the athlete can incorporate into his motor skill. Dr. Loehr suggests that a young player should have many short, concise cue words that accompany forehand, backhand, crosscourt, overhead, and down-the-line shots. These words might be as simple as saying out loud, "footwork, position, footwork." These reminders, over time, become internalized so that the athlete never thinks about the placement of feet in relation to timing of the racket swing. It becomes automatic and programmed into the neuromuscular response.

Different kinds of self-talk and affirmation are geared to the nature of the sport or physical activity. During a marathon race, for example, Olympian Moore would have used a different set of strategies than tennis star Sampras would during his match. A runner, for instance, may choose the word "steady" or the phrase "keep your pace" during races. Likewise, Olympic champion diver Greg Louganis would have used different self-talk reminders than two-time Olympic medalist figure skater Nancy Kerrigan. One athlete might have the luxury of pausing, reflecting, and conducting the self-talk and affirmation imagery, while another may have to use continuous talk and affirmation strategies. Concentration and control may not vary according to the sport, but timing and implementation do. (In Part Three of this book, you'll find examples of sport-specific self-talk and affirmation.)

SELF-CONFIDENCE THROUGH SELF-TALK

You can use self-talk and affirmations to correct improper form and bad habits in a number of sport-related movements. Consider tennis doubles great Gigi Fernandez, who struggled with staying focused, disciplined, and on top of her game during her professional career. She was notorious for inconsistent hitting, poor shot selection, and erratic serves and volleys. Julie Anthony, PhD, her former coach and a former tennis pro, designed specific self-talk exercises on a computer that helped Fernandez stay cool, relaxed, and in control of her game. Using verbal cues to remind Fernandez to stay loose in the knees and relaxed with her forehand shot and during follow-through on her overhead, Dr. Anthony set in motion a series of self-improvement exercises that contributed to Fernandez's gaining greater self-confidence and control of her tennis game.

Probably the most important things to remember about self-talk and using affirmations for building confidence are to stay in the present, stay focused only on the goals at hand, and concentrate. Admittedly, this is easy to say and difficult to do. If we focus too much attention on ourselves and become preoccupied with our own needs, anxiety creeps in, and we worry about every detail. These details often lead to an overconsuming fear that we don't feel quite right or that the weather and temperature are not what we expected.

These thoughts lead to negative emotions that take us away from the present competition. When this happens, small errors in our performance escalate into big ones, and we tend to overreact, leading to more errors and mental mistakes. Thoughts and statements such as "I never compete well in Stuttgart," "I never do well against the Russians," "I don't like the feel of those parallel bars at that gym," or "I never did like the lighting in that rink" can all sabotage a perfect performance.

The trick is to recognize this self-defeating pattern and reprogram the internal dialogue to positive statements. If you don't have a coach, you'll have to listen to yourself carefully and deliberately change the message you're sending to yourself if it's a negative one. Once you are able to find and shift these statements and affirmations and their associated feelings, emotions, and sport behaviors, you'll find yourself reacting with a new confidence and self-esteem.

Leann Warren, a 1980 Olympian, had to leave track and field because of recurring injuries that led to debilitating knee surgery. Yet she readily made the transition into cycling, where she had early, tremendous success. She once noted that she transferred the memories, positive affirmations, and supreme confidence from her track days into cycling. "I had some unfinished business with my track career," Warren explained at the time. "It ended much too early without my fulfilling some important career goals. Consequently, I am taking that unfinished energy, imagery, self-talk, and wonderful confidence and carrying it into my new sport. Even though I am struggling with the nuances of competitive cycling, my confidence is high, and I am able to recall positive thoughts and emotions from my other life."

As we get older and switch from one sport to another, most of us will call up images, self-talk, and levels of confidence that will assist us in our new endeavors. The process of self-talk leading to self-confidence is a lifelong event that we never lose. Instead, we can continually enhance the process.

CHAPTER 4

Clear Your Mind with Breathing and Meditation

Try an experiment. Hold your breath for 30 seconds. Then let go. Repeat this three times. Feel the tightness in your neck, shoulders, and chest. Obviously, you're not going to perform your best feeling like this. Can you imagine Olympic gold medalist Mike Eruzione going through a hockey game with this type of muscle constraint?

Proper breathing not only relaxes you, but it also enhances performance by oxygenating the blood and energizing your brain, nerves, and muscles. Short, shallow breaths from the upper chest constrict your chest muscles; breathing is stressed, inefficient, and labored and not conducive to top athletic effort. In contrast, deep breathing, using the diaphragm, is de-stressing and more efficient. The diaphragm—the muscle between the lungs and abdomen—is the epicenter for proper breathing activity and control. When we inhale, the diaphragm (if it is working correctly) should move down slightly, causing the abdomen to move out and allowing the lungs to expand. This action fills the lungs from the bottom as opposed to the top.

Probably the most important single aspect of staying focused in sport is breathing. Without proper breathing, even the best-conditioned athletes can get easily winded and fatigued and perform poorly. Many young athletes get so aroused before an event that they hyperventilate and then struggle during the competition. This state of overarousal can not only distract the player from the event but also lead to physical unpleasantness such as cramps and vomiting.

Regardless of the sport, most coaches emphasize the importance of proper breathing before motor skill development. It reduces stress and anxiety and increases performance. But athletes don't always take the time to use proper breathing strategies, especially in competitive situations. Yet proper breathing is vital to helping athletes relax and focus—and stay relaxed and focused—for competition.

AN ANTIDOTE FOR COMPETITIVE STRESS

Checking out your breathing before any athletic event should be as routine as making sure that your shoes are tied. Without full, open breathing, you won't be able to perform up to your potential. Breathing properly is important because it sets the stage for other mental and physical responses that cue your body to prepare for competitive stress. With each inhalation, you should induce a feeling of relaxation; with each exhalation, focus on letting go of any muscular tension in the body.

Unfortunately, when we are stressed, as we are during a competitive situation, the natural physiological reaction is to breathe rapidly and shallowly. This can cause problems, because it not only restricts motion but also leads to early fatigue.

Fortunately, athletes and coaches can easily diagnose such a problem and make some dramatic changes. Here's a wonderful exercise used by the late Dorothy Harris, PhD, who was a professor of sport psychology at Pennsylvania State University in University Park, that you can practice in your home or even at the office to improve your breathing technique.

Step 1. Imagine that your lungs have three parts: a lower, middle, and upper section. Now close your eyes and imagine that you are just going to fill up the bottom, or lower, third of your lungs as you breathe in. Do this by imagining that you are pushing out your diaphragm, stretching it to its max, and then opening up your abdomen.

Step 2. Next, imagine filling the second third of your lung cavity. Do this by expanding your chest cavity and raising your rib cage and chest to their maximum capacity.

Step 3. Finally, fill the last sector of your lungs by raising your chest and shoulders.

Do all three stages over and over again with a soft, smooth motion—don't force it. Each time you exhale, remind yourself to pull in your abdominal wall so that all the air is removed from your lungs. And at the end of the exhalation, don't forget to say good-bye to all muscular tension so you feel totally relaxed.

After becoming proficient with this simple exercise, you can expand the program from 30 to 40 deep breaths each day. Each time you practice, close your eyes and visualize the flow of air and energy moving in and out of your system. You can set up little environmental cues throughout your routine to remind yourself when and how to breathe. When the phone rings, when you take a break from working at your computer, when you are in line at the cafeteria, or when you are just getting ready for bed, practice this full, relaxed diaphragm breathing. These cues will be good reminders for more stressful times when you will need to call up your new technique.

You may want to perform breathing exercises while listening to music—something that many athletes do. Often a piece of classical music can set the stage for easy, comfortable, and relaxed breathing. The rhythm of music may allow a person to synchronize his heart with his necessary breathing pace. It is not uncommon to see Jennifer Capriati or Andy Roddick at a tennis match listening to their CD or MP3 players getting the right beat going to tune them up. They are checking in with their breathing and getting their moods in sync with their strategies for the day's competition. Former NBA all-star Patrick Ewing of the New York Knicks has often told sports writers that he doesn't want to be disturbed before a game.

"One hour before the game, I pick a corner of the locker room, put on my headphones, and go into that sacred space," Ewing told a reporter. "Here, I get ready for the matchup; I check out the whole system with my music, while breathing, and focus for the game."

SEE YOURSELF SUCCEED

Many athletes can be seen taking that extra special diaphragm relaxation breath at key moments during competition. Tennis star Gabriela Sabatini is very careful to breathe deeply and fully each time she prepares to serve.

Basketball player Allen Iverson pauses and takes at least two full breaths at the free throw line. Diver Greg Louganis waited (sometimes seemingly forever) at the beginning of his dives to breathe fully before taking the plunge. Skiers Phil and Steve Mahre always took a few extra deep breaths at the starting gates of their giant slalom runs. Lynn Jennings always waits patiently at the start of her cross-country races with a few extra diaphragm breaths. It is a relaxation technique and also a message to the rest of the body that you are now ready to compete.

When you learn to breathe properly and with some degree of control, you breathe more deeply and rhythmically. When you pair increased breathing with an image such as a beautiful gazelle gracefully racing across the plains, you can see, feel, and hear the strength of the breath and the positive energy that goes with it. When breathing techniques become second nature, it's time to learn how to pair appropriate images with inhalation and exhalation exercises.

Ask yourself what images you associate with your sport. Do you use an image of explosiveness, such as coming out of the blocks for the 100 meters? What images might two-time Olympic gold medalist Michael Johnson use? Do your images reflect a graceful motion of twists, turns, and double axels? What are the images that figure skater Sasha Cohen sees before entering the ice rink? What are the images of Olympic cyclist Rebecca Twigg during a closely contested pursuit race? Think about your sport and try to imagine the appropriate images paired with the type of breathing you would like to be doing.

THE KEY TO INNER CALM

Meditation is a form of relaxation, a sort of mental technique that uses the mind to quiet the muscles. It uses a single word, or mantra, that does not possess any meaning or particular significance. In fact, the mantra is intended to be a simple reminder to keep your mind free and clear, yet focused and attentive. The purpose of meditation is to get you passively relaxed, yet still positively focused. The philosophy behind meditation is to quiet the mind, reduce external stimulation, and allow the body to get in sync with a relaxed focus.

When competitors meditate, they shut out the external world and allow only one thought or object to enter their minds, reducing any extra stimulation that might interfere with their quiet time. When athletes meditate, or plug into a singular focus, they allow a passive attitude to take shape.

The feeling is one of "letting it happen" while relinquishing all control of the outside world. If you repeat a phrase such as "easy does it" or "doing fine," you can help your mind reach a calm, nonarousal state, letting all the other thoughts pass without getting distracted. Marathoners, for example, often select a phrase or word that they repeat before the race to help them relax and during the race to help them concentrate and ignore distractions.

Meditation has been used for centuries by practitioners in Eastern cultures. Meditation techniques have been scientifically tested and shown beyond a reasonable doubt to quiet the central nervous system, according to Herbert Benson, PhD, of Harvard Medical School. For years, researchers such as Dr. Benson all across the United States have measured brain wave activity at different stages of meditation focus. In fact, during his keynote address to the American Psychological Association in Chicago in the summer of 2002, Dr. Benson had us all close our eyes and take a few deep breaths. We all got very mellow—a new experience for some in the audience. Tests performed with an electroencephalograph (EEG) have documented that when meditational calmness is reached, brain wave activity shifts from beta, our normal daily operational mode, to alpha, a more relaxed and slowed brain wave.

For people who have achieved a high degree of relaxation, a brain wave shift might take place from alpha to theta, an advanced stage with the mind almost totally inactive. And people with extreme levels of proficiency may move into the trancelike stage of delta. These later two stages are achieved mainly by those who have studied and practiced meditation for many years, such as Eastern yogis.

Experts at the Menninger Foundation in Topeka, Kansas, have conducted research on meditation and brain wave activity for nearly 40 years. They have concluded that one of the most versatile things about meditation is that you can do it anywhere, anytime. This includes meditating just moments before an athletic competition. Many athletes choose to meditate during downtime while on a bus or plane or en route to a competition. This helps them stay calm and get more rest, and it lets them prepare for their events in a relaxed, passive mode.

THE PILATES OPTION

Adding to the new repertoire of game prep, stretching, and mind-body awareness is Pilates, a unique form of physical exercise that involves a combination of resistance training, stretching, and mental concentration. My daughter Shoshana did a bit of research on Pilates training and its origins. She has been a student of Pilates work for the past 6 years.

Devotees of Pilates swear by its ability to strengthen and tone muscles while improving flexibility and posture and increasing awareness of the body. Many recreational athletes (and elite competitors) claim that Pilates has helped them lose weight and tone their muscles, without having to lift weights or do an excessive amount of cardiovascular exercise.

Although Pilates did not surface into the fitness mainstream until the 1990s, the method was developed in the early 1900s. The creator, Joseph H. Pilates, struggled with various physical ailments as a child growing up in Germany. In an attempt to strengthen his own body, Pilates developed a way to rehabilitate himself by using the concept of "muscle control." He further developed the Pilates method when he worked as an orderly in the First World War. In order to recondition soldiers who were wounded in battle, Pilates attached metal springs to hospital beds, which allowed the injured patients to begin using their bodies even before they could walk again. Pilates and the doctors found that the wounded patients who used the technique were healing at an increased rate.

In 1926, Pilates moved to New York City with his wife and opened the first "Pilates" studio. At first, the method was known only by athletes and dancers as a way to rehabilitate after an injury. By the 1950s, dancers like Martha Graham and George Balanchine introduced Pilates to the ballet world. Today, the original Pilates philosophy has been modified into various new methods of exercise that use the "Pilates" name and have adopted the same basic principles. Pilates is used all over the world by ballet dancers, actors, professional athletes, spa centers, and certified trainers at health clubs and studios. And increasingly, the Pilates techniques are being implemented in high schools, club programs, and NCAA arenas as well as among Olympic hopefuls.

SHAKE OFF TENSION

With proper breathing techniques, you can learn any number of meditational strategies that will quiet the mind and enhance performance. Breathing is the first step to recognizing your level of arousal and is an excellent gauge for you to check every morning when you first get up. If your chest feels tight and you feel short of breath early in the day, it might mean that stress and anxiety from a sleepless night are getting the better of you. Once you become more attuned to your breathing, meditation can help you relax.

One of the more positive long-term outcomes of learning meditation and the skill of being passively detached is carrying this skill into your sport. We often see golfers get angry with themselves after hitting a terrible shot, causing a chain reaction of emotions that immediately reminds the muscles to tighten for the next shot. Then the vicious cycle begins again: bad shot, frustration, catastrophic thought, tight muscles, more bad shots, and so on. Any Sunday afternoon during basketball season, we can see the television cameras catch an NBA star shooting a poor free throw, followed by scowling or punching angrily at the air. This sets off a chain reaction from the mind to the muscles that usually carries a message of gloom and doom.

Learning to be focused, yet passively involved, allows you to get rid of negative emotions and muscle memories and to reorient after a bad shot. Sometimes you might hear one athlete yell to another, "Hey, shake it off. Let's get back in the game." This is a cue—a reminder—to let go, be momentarily passive, disengage, and put the bad shot out of your mind. Clear your mind and get on with it.

Breathing and meditation are useful strategies for clearing the mind and getting on with it; together they slow down and reverse the arousal process. Before competition, athletes usually feel a certain amount of excitement in anticipation of the athletic event. Small amounts of arousal and pregame stimulation are healthy and necessary to get ready for the game. Often, however, the arousal seems to overflow, causing butterflies, headaches, cramps, and thoughts laced with negativity. Learning proper counterarousing techniques such as deep breathing and meditation can get you properly tuned up without all the unpleasant side effects. Breathing control can help reduce anxiety as well as produce energy.

TRANSFORM "NERVES" INTO ENERGY

The basic elements to beginning a successful meditation program are simple. First you need to find a quiet, comfortable environment. Next find a mantra—a word or simple phrase that will not arouse you but let you stay calm and focused on a singular task. This might be a word such as "calmness." Some athletes like the words "flow" or "zone."

Repeat the mantra over and over with your eyes closed and your breathing full and deep. If your mind wanders, don't fight the thoughts that seem to pass through; gently allow the distractions to take place and gracefully remind yourself of the chosen word or phrase.

You also need to relax, but relax passively. This simply means that you should not force thoughts or actions, but take a very laissez-faire ("let it happen") attitude. If a negative thought or emotion comes into your mind—such as a past poor performance—let it be. Don't argue with yourself or fight the unpleasant feelings. Let the thought or emotion pass, and passively return to the central focus of your mantra. Last, be sure to stay physically comfortable while you practice your meditation. If you find yourself cramping or getting into awkward positions, shift your body weight.

Initially, the practice of meditation takes some time and commitment. You must first find a quiet place away from the hustle and bustle of an active life and allow yourself time out to practice. Often meditation requires practice of 30 minutes twice a day to get into the flow of this relaxation training. After a few weeks, however, you can meditate 20 minutes once each day, and the acquired relaxation responses will kick in quite naturally.

The important thing to remember is that meditation is passive. You cannot force the relaxation from mind to body. You must simply let it happen. When you repeat your mantra, it is important to stay completely focused on that one word.

When you get to the stage where the mantra is automatic, breathing is full, and the mind is at rest, various body responses occur. With complete meditational focus, an athlete sends signals from the mind through the neural pathways to the muscles and organs, reminding them to stay cool and calm. The body gets shut down by delightful signals being passed along the central nervous system. These signals from the brain tell all messengers throughout the anatomy that all is well at headquarters. This response, caused by a singular focus on breathing and the mantra, removes any negative stimuli and distractions from your system. The previous arousal is reduced to just a passing thought.

By having a strong repertoire of relaxed breathing with meditational techniques, any athlete can switch gears and call into play more oxygen, greater blood supply, enhanced energy reserves, and the appropriate visual cues to supplement athletic strategy. By practicing these techniques in advance, we build in greater awareness of the unexpected and enhance our confidence levels under the stress of competition. Great athletes such as tennis star Steffi Graf, Olympic swimmer and multiple gold-medal winner Janet Evans, and pole vaulter Sergei Bubka always carry with them a visual image, a cognitive cue, and a source of extra energy. They know that they can call up an image, trigger a word or phrase, and get that extra breath when they need it. These are the same athletes who convert negative experiences such as anger, frustration, and aggression to positive moments of arousal with extra oxygen and energy at the finish. These are the winners!

CHAPTER 5

Maximize Performance with Mental Snapshots

Earl Bell, four-time Olympic pole vaulter and bronze medalist in the 1984 Los Angeles Olympics, tells a wonderful story about imagery and mental rehearsal. "I used to train in the winter, and we'd go to this indoor gym that was the same place our basketball team played. Part of our warmup was to shoot some one-on-one and have some fun. My little 3-year-old would come and watch us. A few months later, his grandma bought him a little basketball and a net—a little 4-foot-high goal that had a little ball about 5 inches in diameter, so it fit nicely in his hands. She set up the hoop and put the ball in his hands, and he started to take a shot. But first he squared up in front of the hoop, flipped his wrist, and just took this beautiful little jump shot. This is the first time he had ever played ball. All he'd ever done was watch us, and already he has a great jump shot."

Without realizing it, Bell's youngster had mastered the fundamentals of imagery practice. By watching and visualizing his dad, he had learned a terrific jump shot.

When you think about a typical training regimen for the elite athletes, things such as stopwatches, diets, weights, early morning workouts, and fierce competition will likely spring to mind. You're less likely to think of armchair exercises with athletes sitting quietly and visualizing their competitive strategies. The image of track stars Jackie Joyner-Kersee or Edwin Moses sitting in their easy chairs with their eyes closed is unlikely to be the first to pop into your head when asked to picture what their workouts are like. Obviously, the majority of the elite athlete's training time is, and should be, devoted to physical conditioning. However, mental training by elite athletes is becoming increasingly popular and is now being embraced by coaches, trainers, and sports medicine professionals across the country.

If you were to talk to a number of great athletes, especially from the 1950s, 1960s, and 1970s—before mental training programs were popular in the United States—they would tell you wonderful and creative stories of how they imaged and visualized their success in sport. When my colleague and good friend, the late Bruce Ogilvie, PhD, of San Jose State University in California, started to document and write about this phenomenon, most sports consultants noted that this technique was something they had heard about but didn't have enough hard data to understand how it worked. Dr. Ogilvie knew from his experience as a consultant to many professional teams, including the Los Angeles Lakers and the Portland Trail Blazers, that Americans were 25 years behind the learning curve. Russian and Eastern European athletes had been teaching mental practice—both imagery and visualization strategies—to both coaches and athletes for years.

VISIONS OF VICTORY

Imagery is a very deep, focused type of mental practice. Researchers know that some athletes are able to imitate the actions of others because their minds take mental snapshots of the activities, and then they use these mental pictures as models for their performances. Does this work in recreational sports as well as in competitive situations, including the corporate arena? The answer is definitely yes—and here is why.

Essentially, imagery is the process of receiving information through all of our senses from the external environment. However, images can also be generated as information from our own memories, so that we create our own internal environments or personally enhanced images. Thus, the combination of these two environments, both the imagined and the real-life ones, has a very powerful effect on our nervous systems. Certainly, in most sports, we take in both the internal environment and the intensity of the external environment as well.

You can conceptualize the imagery process by thinking about your home video or DVD player. Your brain acts as its own unique VCR unit, scanning for images and sensory input before they are collected and shuttled onto your mental picture screen. Unlike the VCR/DVD hardware from the department store, your internal equipment—when trained and used properly—will recall with ease feelings, sounds, and smells as well as visual images.

The use of imagery is not a magic bullet but a technique that is used by athletes with great success, frequently and often. As most athletes explain it, imagery is a technique that programs the human mind to respond in a certain way in certain situations. All of us, whether recreational or elite-level athletes, can use imagery to improve our performances. As Olympic ski racer Picabo Street says, "It would be extremely difficult to race downhill at 88 miles per hour without a mental blueprint of very specific images of the course." And, as many Olympians note, to use the psychological skill of imagery and use it correctly, you must practice it in a systematic way.

HOW YOUR BRAIN TAKES A PICTURE

Research in brain physiology has uncovered some startling clues to how imagery functions. The clues have led scientists to vast regions of the brain that control memory, pictures, and vision. Martha Farah, PhD, a professor of psychology at the University of Pennsylvania in Philadelphia, notes that "mental capacities such as memory, perception, imagery, language, and thought processes are rooted in complex structures in the brain." Her research suggests that imagery is not part of language symbols but is simply the chemistry of the visual system.

Using the technology of computerized axial tomography (CAT) and positron-emission tomography (PET), Dr. Farah and other neuropsychologists who examine brain-damaged patients have found that the brain uses the same pathways for seeing as it does for imaging. Here is how it works. When we see something, the image of the object travels into the retina, then to the visual cortex, and then to the higher centers of the brain until it is recognized.

Imagery, in a sense, is "seeing things in reverse." The process begins at the higher centers of the brain and is then passed down to the visual cortex, where it is recognized.

Let's get a clearer picture of the anatomy of your imagery system. When you look at a basketball hoop from a distance of 30 feet, light reflects off the hoop, hits the retina in both of your eyes, and is sent via nerve fibers to a visual holding station in your brain. In the holding station, the image of the hoop is mapped onto the surface of brain tissue just as it appears in the outside world. This holding station is like a movie screen that can display pictures from your eyes or pictures from your memory. The basketball hoop sits in the holding station for a brief time while it is analyzed to determine its edges, contour, color, depth, and many other features.

At this stage, however, your brain doesn't quite realize that the image is a basketball hoop. The analysis must continue. Distinct features of the hoop are sent to two higher brain systems for further analysis. These systems are known as the "what" and "where" systems. The brain needs to match the patterns and shapes of the basketball hoop with other information, such as memory and knowledge of these things, so it goes through a database search to find out what is stored in your mind about basketball.

The temporal lobe is the "what" system, and it has a database that contains thousands of files on shapes and colors. The "where" system is found in the parietal lobe, and it contains a database for location. This area of the brain guides us in knowing distance and depth of field and acts as radar for knowing where things are. When the "what" and "where" databases are being searched, they often combine efforts and go to a third database known as associative memories. This database is like a CD-ROM, with tons of data and files on visual memories.

It is here that a likely good match of identity can be made. Here, the brain puts the "what" and "where" clues together to make a positive recognition of the basketball hoop. If recognition cannot be made, there is one more stop: the mother of all databases, the frontal lobe of the brain. This is considered the highest and most advanced area for decision making. Here you have many indexes, bibliographies, more CD-ROMs, and additional files stored that assist you in deciding what you are looking at.

The importance of this brain mapping has led to some exciting discoveries about imagery. As visual signals from frontal lobes, "what" and "where" lobes, and associative memory lobes send information in one direction; visual signals also send information in the other direction. That is, information is flowing in both directions at all times. The key point here is that imagery is the result of this two-way communication street. So instead of processing visual information from the outside, a visual signal is processed from within. This is the essence of mental imagery.

HOW VISUAL SIGNALS
AFFECT SPORTS PERFORMANCE

Let's try an experiment. Sit quietly for a moment and imagine a soccer ball. Images are stored in your memory on the hard drive in associative memory (one part of the brain), so you do a quick scan and find a general image of a soccer ball. Once found, this image is laid out on your screen in the visual cortex.

Now decide if the ball is rubber or leather. Your mind now shifts to a new database to get more detailed and perhaps more complex information about the soccer ball. This information is found and then shot up to the screen for an imprint. Next, look to see if the ball has writing on it and how large the writing is. Again, a new database search, a find, and a signal shot to the visual cortex for imprint. Job well done!

Using the technology of PET, scientists have speculated that it takes about 1/100,000 of a second to search each database in the brain. Now that is a fast processing chip and a very speedy computer! The most advanced research in this area resulted from studies of people with disabilities and brain damage. According to Dr. Farah, brain-damaged patients often have to conduct dual searches of their brains to find the right answers. A stroke patient, for example, who loses the ability to see colors also can no longer see these colors in his mind. A person with epilepsy who has surgery to reduce seizures is not able to image objects or have any depth of field. Some individuals can have one system intact while another is destroyed. One man who had a brain injury could not tell the color of oranges but knew exactly the distance between New York and California. It's also clear from this research that in healthy individuals, those who can image vividly are also very active with these various brain databases.

What does all this mean for athletics and those who practice imagery? It's simple. If we watch Venus Williams hit one of her dynamic overhead tennis shots, we are noting every aspect of that athletic maneuver. That visual signal is sent, coded, and imprinted in the "where" database. It is the same database that gets used throughout our physical and mental practice of tennis. We use the "where" database to direct actual movement and imagined movement. So if we practice on the court, we are actually strengthening the memory of that database. And vice versa. When we practice our imagery and visualization work, we are also giving more access to that memory.

PRACTICE MAKES PERFECT

Imagery practice involves using all the senses to create an experience in the mind. "All the senses" means not only seeing the experience but smelling, tasting, touching, and feeling it as well. The emotions associated with all of these images are also quite important in understanding the power of this technique. In using imagery to help deal with performance anxiety, reduce pain, and control frustration and anger, athletes must be able to create emotions in their minds. If a tennis player is struggling with anger and rage during the heat of a match, for example, one goal of mental rehearsal might be to practice impulse control and anger management so it doesn't interfere with the focus of playing. In practicing imagery, we must be able to use the emotions associated with performance to help us better understand and cope with the competitive experience.

Perhaps some of us are just average weekend skiers. But after watching 1994 Olympic gold medalist Tommy Moe race down the hills of Lillehammer, Norway, or 2002 Olympic medalist Bode Miller in Salt Lake City, we rush outdoors and ski better than we ever thought we could because we are inspired by the style and mobility of these great athletes. We are able to mimic Moe's and Miller's fluid and graceful action on the slopes because our minds take snapshots of the skill and record them in a specific region of our brains. These pictures get called upon over and over—much as we call up information on the hard drives of our personal computers—and act as blueprints for our future performances. Imagery is based on memory, and we constantly reinforce the internal process by a flood of new pictures from external experiences to our minds.

We must also realize that in the process of expanding our repertoire— our imagery database—we can also create new images in our minds by practicing diligently. Danny Everett, 1988 Olympic sprinting gold medalist who set a world record in the 400 meters, uses imagery consistently to reinforce his training.

"Just before practice, I do a certain amount of imagery in preparation for my day of workouts," Everett says. "That way, when I get ready to race, I'm already prepared. The night before competition, I also do imagery and visualization practice so that I can get into the rhythm previously established during my workouts." He can quantify his payoff based on the amount of physical and psychological training he did, including imagery practice.

Everett reminded me that going into his 1990 indoor world record in the 400-meter race in Stuttgart, Germany, he was in the best shape of his life. "During the race I felt like I wasn't even moving fast," he said. "It felt like a comfortable jog around the track. It was easy; there was no struggle, and I felt a floating quality to the race . . . almost like I was in slow motion. I felt like I had been to that race in Stuttgart in those weather conditions in my mind already. I looked up and couldn't believe my time. . . . It didn't feel like a world record." After an important competition, many athletes report this floating, in-sync, effortless quality to their performances. This report is not mystical or even magical, but usually attributed to much practice—much mental practice.

SEE IT, THEN DO IT

The appeal of mental imagery techniques is that we know they work. Not only does research show that imagery works, but numerous athletes swear by it. Granted, we don't hear competitors talking about the impulses-from-the-brain-to-the-muscles theory or the imagery coding system. But we do hear numerous examples of cyclists, skiers, runners, tennis players, volleyball players, swimmers, weight-lifting athletes, and others who testify to the extraordinary power of this form of mental rehearsal.

When I first met Sergei Bubka in person, at a press conference outside the Olympic stadium in Barcelona, several of the international media asked him how he trains for his pole vault competitions. He told all of us (in perfect English) that he uses a lot of imagery and visualization when practicing, both on and off the field. "I hang out in the gym and train with the Russian gymnasts who are renowned for their use of mental practice techniques," he explained to me back in 1992. We met again in Copenhagen at an International Olympic Committee meeting (he now serves as an athlete advisor) in March of 2003, and I reminded him of our conversation. He told me that he still stays in shape and trains in the same fashion.

As Bubka described his daily workouts, he spoke in terms of internal and external images as well as visual and feeling senses. His words that day reminded me of the studies about the success of competitive gymnasts who use a great deal of internal imagery. How we see things in our mind's eye may vary from person to person, but all of us have the potential to enhance imagery the more we practice it.

And still others use imagery but just don't call it that. Julie Anthony, PhD, tennis pro turned clinical psychologist, believes that nearly all athletes have their own forms and styles of mental rehearsal. "They have their own techniques, and they choose not to put titles or clinical labels on them," she explains.

In my days as a college gymnast at the University of Texas in the 1960s, the term "mental practice" was not part of my athletic or academic vocabulary. I don't ever remember hearing coaches or athletes speak about a "visualization strategy." But unconsciously, we all took our training and required routines home with us and practiced them throughout our waking (and nocturnal) hours. It was something we did, but most of us didn't really know that the process was happening.

YOU CAN CALL THE SHOTS

The ability to control imagery is a significant advantage when you're preparing for athletic competition. Athletes say that controlling the pictures on your own internal screen before you get out on the field is very useful. Because practice makes perfect, you should always practice the correct imagery response. Remember that practice also makes imperfect if you are practicing the wrong imagery response. In tennis, as in any other sport, strong emotions are involved in the mental practice of the correct athletic skills. When you are tense or angry, you might fire off an out-of-control backhand followed by a series of terrible shots. If you don't correct the imagery, the shots get worse.

Imagery and other forms of mental practice play major roles in the performance of sport. According to Dr. Anthony, some athletes will not accept the notion of imagery as a training strategy. "Some of my tennis players are so rebellious that if you call it mental rehearsal or visualization training, they resist. So I just expose certain rebels to our more grounded tennis professionals—give them a taste of a positive role model. When they get exposed to a Martina and her mental and psychological work ethic, it just tends to rub off naturally."

Unfortunately, the message of good, solid training preparation, both physiological and psychological, doesn't often occur until the last minute. Often competitors will try to implement mental practice skills the week before a big competition. This is difficult to do for two reasons. First, just as you train your physical skills, you must train your mind with imagery skill development. This takes time and much practice; it doesn't happen overnight.

The second problem with eleventh-hour mental training practice is that some athletes experience major arousal and anxiety before competitions. Many athletes get performance anxiety 5 to 7 days before a major competition. This causes changes in sleeping and eating patterns and disrupts the emotional state. You need mental training techniques to calm you down at this point, but while you're in this jittery, pre-event state is no time to learn these techniques. As a college gymnast, I remember not sleeping well or not sleeping at all days before a major dual meet. Before going to the Southwest Conference Championship, my eating, sleeping, and brain functions seemed to be completely out of rhythm. Too bad that we didn't know more about relaxation and mental practice skills back in the 1960s. The Longhorns may have had better outcomes.

CHAPTER 6

Relax to Cool Down—
And Rev Up

Relaxation is a key to physical and mental skill development. Look at 1980 and 1984 Olympic gymnasts Julianne McNamara and Kathy Johnson.

McNamara, who won a gold and two silver medals at the 1984 Olympics, was so proficient on the uneven bars that she developed a technique that was named after her. And visualization and relaxation played roles in its development.

"I think the reason that the McNamara Mount came about was that I saw it happen way before it developed into a gymnastic trick," she explained. "I was very relaxed and able to visualize the trick before getting on the bars and doing it. After practicing it in my mind, it seemed quite fluid and easy when I got to actually perform it."

Her teammate, Johnson (now Johnson-Clarke and a dear friend of mine), who won silver and bronze medals in 1984, tells an unusual story about using imagery and visualization after a long relaxation session.

"I was competing in Europe at an international meet, and I wanted to do something special for my floor routine," says Johnson. "I didn't change my actual physical routine, but emotionally and spiritually, I wanted to express myself differently in my gymnastics that day. My life had gone through some dramatic changes, and I wanted to express some of my personality and my struggle in my floor exercise. I felt very emotional; the images and visualizations were very strong going into the event, and I remember being very relaxed. I scored very well, but more importantly, I felt this major emotional release after the routine. My brother called me later to say that he saw my gymnastic competition on television in the United States. He said that he saw something very dramatic happening out there, as if my life had been transformed, and I was telling a story. It still leaves me with chills today when I tell people."

MORE THAN JUST CHILLING OUT

In trying to better understand the relationship between imagery and visualization skills and enhanced performance, we need to stop, rewind the tape a few frames, and look carefully at how best to achieve this. When social psychologist Jacqueline Golding, PhD, and I interviewed elite track and field athletes about their use of mental practice, one question kept emerging in our research: How do athletes achieve mental comfort levels that allow them to use imagery and visualization strategies effectively?

The answer, we found, is in relaxation. In interviews of elite athletes that we conducted, nearly all the Olympic competitors said that they had to achieve a state of relaxation to be able to practice effective imagery and visualization skills. Dr. Golding and I were struck by how many successful athletes practiced some form of relaxation techniques on a regular basis—in some cases, seven times a week. These techniques always included a form of deep breathing exercises and were often supplemented with recorded music or a tape of waves gently hitting the seashore.

Many athletes will tell you that they do not practice a formal relaxation procedure such as meditation, but they design their own deep-breathing relaxation procedures to meet their own needs. Some athletes have experimented with transcendental meditation, a process that combines deep breathing with differential muscle relaxation strategies. Other competitors just go to a favorite chair when they're tight and wound up, close their eyes, and breathe deeply to settle the butterflies.

One of the major lessons that I have learned from 25 years of working with elite athletes, however, is that relaxation is just one ingredient in the delicate recipe for enhanced performance. Yes, it is important, but it cannot work alone. Relaxation must be used in conjunction with imagery and visualization training. I underscore this because often coaches will say to their young competitors, "Just relax, chill out, and you will perform well."

For a handful of athletes, this simple advice may work. But for the majority of competitors, whether at the middle school, college, Olympic, professional, or masters level, just "chilling out" won't cut it. Relaxation must be cultivated via a structured training program that includes imagery and visualization strategies.

FEWER DISTRACTIONS MEAN SHARPER FOCUS

What we know about mental practice and relaxation training today is quantum leaps beyond what we knew in the 1960s. When preparing a mental practice training program, we prepare ourselves for the actual event as well as all the emotions that surround that athletic experience. Most of us are susceptible to all sorts of emotions, including anxiety, and emotions can be very disruptive to learning and practicing imagery skills.

Relaxation is extremely useful for athletes such as gymnasts, who find it particularly important to reduce arousal before competition. For one thing, they have to compete on one apparatus while other events are occurring simultaneously. Gymnastics also requires delicate timing, balance, strength, agility, and tremendous concentration all at the same moment. The slightest distraction, muscle tightness, or mental lapse can lead to a mistake, fall, point reduction, and perhaps even serious injury. So staying calm, mentally and physically, is doubly important.

Learning how to relax will help you to practice imagery and visualization. Sometimes, however, the reverse is true. If you're adept at imagery and other forms of mental rehearsal, then it may be easier to relax. If, for example, you can visualize your favorite beach with sky-blue water and soft, fine-grain sand, then this visual image of a warm, sunny place might introduce a feeling of complete relaxation and a sense of calmness.

Relaxation to enhance visualization is analogous to fine-tuning your VCR or DVD when you have interference and static lines on the screen. You are attempting to clean up the picture so that the resolution is pure and focused—in sync with the images projected from the tape or disc. Your mind is like the VCR/DVD: The signals are always strong, but occasionally, stray thoughts and negative signals cause fuzziness on your mental picture screen. This interrupts the clarity of your image from the memory area of your brain. So when you do relaxation techniques, you're essentially fine-tuning the wave band. Athletes who do much imagery work tell us that they can go immediately into their mind's eye to a stadium or race course and give vivid details of the terrain, contours of the surface, weather and sky conditions, and even dew point or moisture in the air. These are finely tuned athletes with very efficiently operating internal VCR/DVD units.

A LESSON IN LOOSENING UP

One of the most studied and practiced forms of relaxation that is often used for imagery enhancement is progressive relaxation, a method of tensing and relaxing one muscle group at a time, from head to toe. Often called PR, progressive relaxation was developed in the 1930s by Edmund Jacobson, MD, of the University of Chicago. The techniques have been used all over the world and for many disciplines, including athletic performance. The Jacobson progressive relaxation techniques have been useful for people suffering from major illness or those recovering from surgery. Women in Lamaze childbirth classes also use these techniques to prepare for labor.

Many athletes practice progressive relaxation before and after competition. Some just practice it whenever they have free time. Athletes often travel long distances by car, bus, and plane and become stiff and cramped when they can't get enough blood and oxygen to their muscle groups. Progressive relaxation often alleviates some of that distress. Often, when muscles are already tight or sore from a practice or a long workout, this may take longer, but the benefit will be greater relaxation in that muscle group.

Cyclists, including six-time Tour de France winner Lance Armstrong, often report that after 4 to 5 hours of hard hill-climbing, progressive muscle relaxation is essential to bring back normal feeling and muscle control in overstressed quadriceps. Cliff Stenquist, a prominent cyclist, skier, and massage therapist, notes that you have to find the balance. "When you are sprinting on the bike or on a Nordic trail, you are depleting the oxygen and glycogen supplies," he says. "This can lead to major cramps, increased tension, and sore muscles. You have to take care of your body, evaluate the parts that get stressed, and then do some major relaxation work to get ready for the next workout."

To learn to enhance proper imagery and visualization skills with relaxation, you need a quiet place away from the training venues and gyms with their external distractions. It's best to learn imagery skill development in a quiet, nonthreatening environment so you can practice and master the skill with confidence before you get to a competitive environment. This lets you build a strong repertoire—a focus and concentration with imagery skills— before entering an arena that requires those skills. By removing sights, sounds, noises, and external stimuli, you lower your arousal states, which in turn reduces muscle tightness and negative thoughts so that you're in control of your emotions.

The Jacobson PR technique is quite simple. Sit in a chair and begin to tighten your right hand and fist. After 10 seconds of tightness, release all the muscles and let your hand go completely limp. Now do the same for your left hand, making a tight fist and increasing the muscle tension for 10 seconds. Now release. Notice the tension, followed by a sensation of letting go and relaxed energy flow. It should feel pretty good. You have just begun the first PR session. You can see that if you were to spend 30 to 40 minutes each day tightening and loosening all the major muscle groups of your body, the outcome might be quite delightful. Try it tonight before going to sleep.

Many sports consultants and even athletic stores offer a series of deep-breathing and relaxation tapes to quiet the mind and body. Often a sport psychologist will recommend to an athlete and coach that they create a tailor-made relaxation tape. This tape would include progressive relaxation, with the voice of the coach or athlete reminding the athlete how to relax, how to breathe, and how to use imagery. These have been quite effective for athletes who pair the tape with a structured imagery program, which you can do on your own or with the help of your coach or a sport psychologist.

When I was asked to consult with the US Olympic Fencing Team, I had athletes make tapes using a particular "quieting response." This quieting response was a combination of deep muscle relaxation from head to toe with full and deep breathing techniques that offered a time-out from the rigors and pressures of training. Most of the Olympic fencers who used the tape reported that it gave them a chance (and an excuse) to sit quietly away from the gym and get centered. It was a time-out from training and worrying about competition and a peaceful interlude before going back to the gym.

MONITORING THE MUSCLES AND THE MIND

Relaxation techniques to enhance imagery and visualization strategies stem from two different concepts. The first is the muscle-to-mind relationship, which suggests that athletes can train their muscles to become ultrasensitive to any level of tension and arousal. The purpose in learning this technique is to train the muscles to diagnose the situation, thus becoming aware of any tension and then releasing it immediately.

The second concept is the mind-to-muscle relationship that is usually present in meditation techniques. Here, the athlete becomes aware of arousal and tension first from the mind and then sends the appropriate quieting or tranquility response to the muscles. Both techniques are equally effective and are precipitated by an awareness that allows for any tension to be interrupted in the nerve endings as impulses travel throughout the central nervous system. Whether the nervous energy is traveling to or from the mind is irrelevant. The point is that there is an interruption of this arousal and nervous energy flow so that the message is recoded for relaxation.

This all may sound very neurological and quite technical, but research shows that the techniques for quieting muscle responses are quite simple. Many coaches will begin a workout with muscle-relaxation sessions during warmups and then close out a session with a cooldown of relaxation techniques. By doing the muscle relaxation before and after athletic practice, you are simply reminding the muscles, neurons, and their electronic pathways to be relaxed for the next session. You are, in essence, building in a muscle memory similar to athletic skill development memory.

When you learn to relax completely, you send messages to the entire body, offering a ground rule for how to react in stressful situations. This ground rule sets the stage for moving to imagery and visualization techniques. When you are relaxed, there is no mental, emotional, or cognitive interference. All the airwaves are clear, and it opens up the channels for image clarity and visual fine-tuning.

You can make your own tape. Talk your way through a complete body relaxation. Tell yourself to get comfortable and visualize a pleasant, relaxing image. Then instruct yourself to tighten each muscle group, one by one, and then gradually release the tension, while breathing deeply and fully. Think of this as a sort of dialogue with your body, with imagery as a buffer. The advantage of making your own tape is that you can custom-tailor it by using imagery scenes that you find particularly restful. And taking responsibility for making your own tape may make the tape that much more useful.

The journey to full relaxation often makes it easier to learn skills that might enhance your athletic performance. Many athletes note that when they can get to a quiet, comfortable environment, away from loud music and the hustle of day-to-day life, they often find solace and a natural relaxation environment. When this solitude is not easily accessible, however, it is important to know that you can go inside yourself and find it within.

CHAPTER 7

Improve Your Game with Guided Imagery

At one imagery presentation, I spoke about guided imagery to a group of young gymnasts training for a state championship on the West Coast. I began the lecture by asking this group of 40 competitors to close their eyes and mentally walk through their balance beam routines. I then asked them if they could see their routines clearly in their mind's eye.

To my surprise, all the young athletes in the group not only saw themselves but also heard and felt specific feelings in their bodies as they mentally moved gracefully across the beam. Then the conversation shifted abruptly.

One young lady raised her hand and declared that she felt fear and anxiety in her imagery when she experienced this practice session in her mind. This prompted other competitors to speak up and say they wanted to deal with the apprehension and anxiety of falling, both in competition and in training. Now we had some great material to begin our discussion of guided imagery. Eventually, I was able to help individual competitors reframe or shift their images to more positive outcomes.

Guided imagery practice and training are not only helpful for improving a particular skill but also, as you can imagine, very useful in dealing with fear, anxiety, and too much arousal about the performance goals in general. It is a skill that anyone can learn, practice with ease, and benefit from.

A SKILL ANYONE CAN LEARN

The exciting part of learning the control and perspective that come with vivid imagery practice is that you can use this skill in any individual or team sport throughout your life. An entire basketball team can use guided imagery to help develop and execute plays. By slowing down a half-court offense, the coach can convey an image of how each of the five players can set up the appropriate offense for a score. Likewise, a skier can use a series of guided images and visualizations to help develop a strategy for a giant slalom race.

Numerous elite competitors have used imagery to keep them at the top of their sports. Consider these athletes.

Holly Flanders, Olympic skier and three-time World Cup winner, believes that imagery and visualization training were essential for her to stay in the sport. After some unpleasant spills, she lost confidence and needed the help of a professional consultant to get back on the slopes. Guided imagery that depicted specific visuals and scenes of safety and success on each downhill turn gave her a new lease on her Olympic career.

The late Willie Davenport, a five-time Olympian, said that his imagery and visualization strategies were rather unorthodox, but nonetheless essential tools. As a world-class 110-meter hurdler for more than 20 years, Davenport was able to visualize each opponent in every lane from the moment they entered the blocks.

Jeff Blatnick, a gold-medal wrestler in the 1984 Olympics, used guided imagery during a near-fatal encounter with Hodgkin's disease and lymphoma to help recover and stay physically and mentally tuned up for his matches.

Russ Hellickson, head wrestling coach at Ohio State University in Columbus and two-time Olympic silver medalist, has his athletes perform a unique ritual when they enter and exit his coaching office at the Woody Hayes facility. He requires that each athlete touch a sign on the door that reminds them to be winners. "This is a cue—a constant visual and kinesthetic reminder to each athlete," explains Hellickson. "When they touch that sign, it symbolizes a win for our whole team, and they are reinforcing that thought, feeling, and emotion in their internal imagery." It must work: Hellickson has had terrific success at Ohio State, and many of his athletes have gone on to compete in the Olympics.

Researchers know something of the biophysiology as well as the psychology of visualization techniques and how it serves our minds and bodies. At almost any library in the United States, you can find an extensive body of literature that describes how this technique works, why it works, and how an imagery program can help people both in athletics and in the workplace. What you'll likely have trouble picking up from books in the library, however, is which type of imagery is appropriate specifically for you and your sport.

HOW DO YOU SEE WHAT YOU SEE?

To develop a guided imagery program that will work for you, you must first answer these basic questions.

- How do you experience images?

- Do you perceive an image by sight, hearing, touch, or feel?

- What are the sensory modes that allow you to experience an image?

To help get a perspective on how different people experience images, ask friends or colleagues how they see themselves shooting hoops, hitting tennis shots, or skiing on their favorite mountain. Ask a child to close his eyes and experience an image; ask him to describe his favorite dessert. All of these different perspectives will give you a richer sense of how you and other people sense images.

You need to focus on whether you see, hear, or feel images. Chances are that you do all three. Rainier Martens, PhD, author and pioneer in sport psychology, has designed a wonderful instrument called the Sport Imagery Questionnaire (see page 56) that will help you understand your imagery ability.

You must address three major components of the guided imagery model in any training program. You'll need to learn how to:

- Develop vivid images

- Control those images

- Understand your perspective of imagery

Perspective simply means whether you experience your sport from within, as in the first person, or see yourself from the outside. The

(continued on page 58)

SPORT IMAGERY QUESTIONNAIRE

This questionnaire, developed by Rainier Martens, PhD, author and pioneer in sport psychology, was designed to help you pinpoint how you experience imagery. Follow the instructions and then add your score at the end to determine if you more intensely experience the sights, sounds, feelings, or moods of an image. This knowledge will help you individualize your mental training program. You'll learn to concentrate on those areas you experience the most vividly as you work on controlling or altering your mental images.

Read the questions below and rate each one using the following scale.

1 = no image present

2 = not clear or vivid, but a recognizable image

3 = moderately clear and vivid

4 = clear and vivid

5 = extremely clear and vivid

1. Practicing Alone

Pick one skill in your sport and imagine yourself doing this wherever you normally practice—but with no one else there. Close your eyes for a minute; try to see yourself, hear the sounds, feel your body perform the movement, and be aware of your state of mind.

_____ a. How well did you see yourself doing the activity?

_____ b. How well did you hear the sounds of doing the activity?

_____ c. How well did you feel yourself making the movements?

_____ d. How aware were you of your mood?

2. Practicing with Others

You're doing the same thing, but practicing with the coach and your teammates present. This time you make a mistake that everyone notices. Close your eyes for a minute to imagine making the error and the situation afterward.

_____ a. How well did you see yourself in this situation?

_____ b. How well did you hear the sounds?

_____ c. How well did you feel yourself making the movements?

_____ d. How well did you feel the emotions of the situation?

3. Watching a Teammate

Think of a teammate making a mistake in a critical part of a game or competition, such as missing a goal or falling.

_____ a. How well did you see your teammate?

_____ b. How well did you hear the sounds?

_____ c. How well did you feel your own physical presence or movement?

_____ d. How well did you feel the emotions of the situation?

4. Competing

Imagine yourself performing the same or similar activity in a game or competition, but imagine yourself doing it skillfully with the spectators and teammates showing their appreciation. Close your eyes for about a minute and imagine this situation as clearly as possible.

_____ a. How well did you see yourself in this situation?

_____ b. How well did you hear the sounds in this situation?

_____ c. How well did you feel yourself making the movements?

_____ d. How well did you feel the emotions of the situation?

Scoring

Add up your total score for each a answer, b answer, and so on. Then add all four figures for a total score.

a. Visual (what you saw) _____

b. Auditory (what you heard) _____

c. Kinesthetic (what you felt) _____

d. Mood (how you felt) _____

Total _____

Take a look at where you fall in the imagery zone. Once you have decided where you are, pay attention to how much of your day (both in and out of the gym) involves imagery experiences.

advantage of internal imagery is that you experience yourself performing a skill. External imagery might be similar to taking a movie camera and shooting a practice and then replaying it from the angle of the cameraman. It lets you step back from the experience and be an impartial observer.

Both perspectives are very important strategies in the guided imagery developmental process, and the exercises that follow will help you determine the difference.

DETAILS MAKE VISIONS VIVID

Psychologist Robin Vealey, PhD, has designed exercises to assist athletes with controlling images and making those images more vivid. These exercises will help you with any sport, regardless of your competitive level.

Step 1. Ask a friend to sit in a chair directly in front of you. Close your eyes and try to get a sharp image of this person. Try to visualize details of this person: her face, her hair color, her muscle structure, and her mannerisms. Now imagine that person talking. Try to imagine the sound and the quality of the voice. Imagine her facial expressions. Now think about how you feel about this person as she talks. Check out your emotions about her. Are they feelings of respect, love, anger, intimacy, trust?

Step 2. Sit quietly in your home or office and imagine yourself at your gym or workout center. You might even imagine yourself at a place where you will be competing. The place you have chosen in your mind is empty—vacant, except for you. You are all alone there. Notice how very quiet and peaceful the surroundings are. Now imagine details about this place: how it smells, the height of the ceiling, the temperature, the humidity, the sounds, and the feeling of the floor.

Next, shift the imagery focus to the same place but fill it now with an overflowing crowd. It is competition day, the fans are there to see you compete, and it has a festival-type atmosphere. Notice the sounds, the smells, the surroundings, and the temperature again. As you get ready to compete, notice how you feel. Notice your heart rate, your perspiration, your breathing, and your excitement and arousal levels.

Step 3. For the next guided image, sit quietly and close your eyes. Check out your breathing; it should be from the diaphragm and very deep, full, and relaxed.

Now imagine your sport: diving, swimming, weight lifting, skiing, cycling, or whatever. Mentally go to the place where you perform and pick the first skill that you perform in your sport. Notice how your muscles feel when you get ready to execute this skill. Feel the tension and the excitement in your stomach and your breathing as you perform. Perform this first skill over and over in your mind's eye so that you have a complete picture of every aspect of this skill.

Now think about how flawless you are and the perfection in your performance. Remind yourself that you are like a well-crafted automobile that is in sync at any speed or under any driving conditions.

Go through this skill one more time, emphasizing an awareness of sound, touch, feel, and complete vividness as you perform. You have now achieved a high degree of vivid imagery.

REWIND AND REVIEW

Select a sport and begin mentally practicing it. This can be a sport that you are just learning or one that you might be playing in the NCAA finals. Guided imagery is not an exclusive club for elite athletes; you can use it at any level of proficiency. Now imagine in your mind's eye your breathing and any amount of tension that might exist in your arms and legs.

Notice if you are excited or aroused as you picture your sport. Next start playing and search your memory bank for a competitor or a teammate. Now imagine yourself executing a series of skills with your teammate or against an opponent.

Notice your mistakes. Slow down the picture when you see a mistake, running through each frame in slow motion. Now speed up again to regular pace and continue to play well. If you see or feel yourself making a mistake in your imagery, slow down the visualization, correct the mistake, return to excellent play and speed up the mental tape.

Congratulations! You've just taken control of your imagery in the practice session. It is a fun and creative process. It also works for improving schoolwork, meeting office demands, and addressing issues in your personal life. Try it out in any setting.

VARY YOUR VANTAGE POINT

For this exercise, mentally experience your sporting event as if you were seeing yourself compete from the stands as a spectator. Think of it as if you have a video camera and you're filming yourself for the 11:00 p.m. sports news. Notice how you do. Look objectively at all the movements: How tight you are, how relaxed you become, how your body moves with grace and ease. Now shift the scene and become that person. Go inside the competitor, taking the video camera with you. Now you are shooting the camera from inside yourself; all the moves and motions and tensions are experienced from within, from an internal perspective.

Notice the difference between the spectator view and the internal, first-person view. Notice how you feel and what you experience when you shift from the outside to the inside. Make a mental note of these differences, which may be very dramatic or very subtle. Consider which perspective (internal or external) works best for you. Incidentally, the 1988 US Olympians whom social psychologist Jacqueline Golding, PhD, and I studied used both internal and external imagery to improve their skill levels. Some found it useful to focus from the outside; some preferred the internal mechanism to improve and enhance their performances. There is no right or wrong here; it is merely a matter of knowing which style best fits you.

Once you know about your ability to maintain vividness, control, and perspective, you can spend more time implementing and practicing the guided imagery skill. Coaches, parents, and athletes alike need to remember that there is no magic in building a guided imagery program. It is straightforward, yet you must practice it daily. You need to build it into the physical training program from day one. It should not be an add-on or afterthought, but part of the total training package. (On page 240, you'll find a guided imagery session appropriate for any sport.)

ACCESS YOUR IMAGE BANK

There's one more essential ingredient in successful mental practice training: You have to practice correctly to achieve success. Conversely, if you practice a skill incorrectly in your guided imagery, chances are 99 out of 100 that you will take that imagery practice session into the competitive arena and perform poorly. You need to practice correct form and proper skill development and use the appropriate images that associate with those skills. If this is done correctly in your mind, you can then transfer that skill to the athletic venue.

Guided imagery is like any other skill. Every individual differs in how he accesses visual pictures in his mind and then uses them in daily life. Just as athletes have different abilities to perform various sports, athletes also have strengths and weaknesses in controlling the vividness and clarity of their images with skill enhancement. The good news is that imagery is just like any skill development: The more you practice, the better you get. If you shoot free throws for 2 hours each morning, no doubt you will improve this skill. Likewise, if you practice guided imagery, you will have easier access to those images, and they will assist you during the heat of competition.

The important thing to remember when designing a guided imagery program is that it must fit your style and preference—meaning, how you access your images. Are they mainly sight, sound, or feel or a combination of all three? The ultimate program, of course, would combine all three types, allowing greater imagery control and more effective outcomes with your performance. This goal, however, is not always possible. I remember working with a three-time Olympic fencer, now a prominent fencing coach on the East Coast. He could only hear his images and the sounds of the foil hitting the target. He could not, and would not, see his images when training. Together we developed an audiotape, and it worked out fine. But it was important for both of us to know how he experienced images so that we could build a program that worked for him.

Use the Resources section at the back of this book to find a coach or facilitator who is qualified to assist you in starting a guided imagery program.

CHAPTER 8

Use Visual Rehearsal to Fine-Tune Your Style

At the 1994 Winter Olympics in Lillehammer, Norway, downhill racer and gold medalist Tommy Moe used a series of slow-motion mental images to get a feel for the icy and sometimes treacherous turns on the giant slalom. Picabo Street, silver-medal-winning skier at Lillehammer, also used imagery to analyze and correct errors when preparing for a second run on the downhill racing course. Downhill ski champion Bode Miller reports that in Salt Lake City he used a series of "freeze frame images" to slow down the gravity of the course so that he could navigate with precision skill.

These are components of a procedure known as visual motor behavior rehearsal (VMBR). This is the process of creating a mental video before an event and then using it to analyze and correct errors that may have occurred in both real and imagined events.

Richard Suinn, PhD, emeritus professor of psychology at Colorado State University in Fort Collins, developed this procedure while working with alpine skiers. Dr. Suinn describes it best: "The VMBR technique combines relaxation and imagery in a format that allows individuals to desensitize themselves to a stressful situation."

Some clinical psychologists use this format to help people deal with their fear of heights or snakes or any other phobia. However, Dr. Suinn added an additional component that allows individuals to not only change a particular behavior but also control imagery. Athletes bring the imaged pictures and scenes into focus during the VMBR strategy to improve. These scenes tend to emphasize behaviors that involve physical or psychological skills associated with motor performance.

MENTAL BLUEPRINT FOR WINNING

For the most part, the mental practice of VMBR is aimed at removing unwanted and undesirable movements that affect athletic performance. This technique has been used widely with Olympic and professional athletes to reduce the possibility of poor performance, and it can work for you as well. Many sport consultants and psychologists are hired by professional baseball, football, basketball, and hockey leagues to help athletes to better performances through VMBR techniques. Owners, managers, and coaches depend on these consultants and their interventions to help them produce winning teams. Because professional and Olympic sports are such big business, acquiring the winning edge through enhanced mental practice is a very important process.

The VMBR strategy can be used for different purposes. After an athlete masters the general sense of relaxation and confidence, for instance, VMBR can be used to control tension, rehearse for an upcoming competition, remove stress in parts of the body, and enhance the winning feeling.

You can use VMBR to enhance your ability by imagining yourself performing well and feeling confident as you compete. How does this work? VMBR has four goals.

1. Technique enhancement

2. Error analysis and correction

3. Preparation for competition

4. Skill enhancement

When an athlete such as Michelle Kwan, three-time Olympic figure skater, wants to improve her performance on the ice, for example, she works within a four-step program to look critically at her tricks and maneuvers in her sport. She could use VMBR at any stage of her training to visualize a particular skill on the ice. She could then practice the skill through a series of images and visualizations brought into slow-motion focus and ultimately improve her performance. This is technique enhancement.

Kwan might also use VMBR to analyze and correct errors from falls on the ice; this is error analysis.

Once an athlete identifies the error and corrects it mentally, he is then encouraged to implement these changes on the basketball court, track, tennis court, or ice rink, in the pool, or in any athletic venue. Athletes can use visual motor behavior rehearsal to prepare for competition by imagining the details of the competitive situation and the ways in which they will meet challenges. This is the preparation for competition. The corrected format both on the court and in the mind of the visual athlete becomes critical in preparing for competition.

Skill enhancement comes with practice, and lots of it. Martina Navratilova, Venus and Serena Williams, Jennifer Capriati, and Lindsay Davenport, who go out and hit hundreds of serves day in and day out on the tennis courts, are practicing their enhancement strategies. They have gone to the clubhouse to watch their videos, they've listened to their coaches, and they are now restructuring their strokes and using their mental blueprints to enhance the quality of their tennis serves. This is all part of the VMBR strategy.

GET RID OF NEGATIVE ENERGY

One of the best examples of the power of VMBR occurred in 1983, when a young researcher at the University of North Carolina demonstrated that basketball shooting could improve by 7 percent after practicing this mental technique. The study also found that the players who practiced VMBR also improved their winning streaks significantly. In 1985, a study by Dr. Suinn showed that skilled athletes who practiced VMBR got better, while less-skilled athletes actually did worse after using this mental training.

The trick here is that if you practice the correct response, you improve; if you practice the incorrect response, you might do worse. It's that simple. Athletes with low skill levels might be doing the wrong movement, and by practicing the incorrect mental picture, they distort the blueprint and send the incorrect signals to all the various muscle groups. This eventually leads to poor training and poor skill development. If you have a mediocre jump shot and you correct the jump shot by shooting at the wrong height of your jump, then the result is a messy jump shot.

A 1983 study by W. Timothy Gallwey, best-selling author of *The Inner Game of Golf*, had golfers use the VMBR technique with a proper putting technique. A second group of golfers was told to visualize the incorrect putting technique. The correct group improved dramatically, while the incorrect group of putters did not. In fact, their putting got worse.

In one study with a group of cross-country skiers, researchers used the technique to monitor pain and tension during long and arduous workouts. They instructed the competitive skiers to remove any negative thoughts or preoccupations about the discomfort of the cold and the poor quality of snow. This variation of the VMBR technique was to "thought stop," or control, the negative energy that might lead to a poor performance. Telling yourself bad things such as "The pain is unbearable" may put you in the wrong frame of mind, triggering muscle reactions that might keep you from finishing the race or performing well. In this experiment, thought stopping led to a changed belief system, shifting the focus from discomfort to feeling competent and skiing successfully.

Other studies have trained athletes to deal with cramps, fatigue, exhaustion, and overall distress. These procedures are particularly helpful to marathon runners, who experience all the symptoms mentioned above and often need to disassociate from this agony to focus on a successful race.

A TRIAL RUN

VMBR allows you to experience sensory-motor sensations of an athletic skill that mimic real experiences. Mimicking or practicing these motor skills involves emotional, physiological, and kinesthetic experiences. Let's walk through a quick VMBR practice session.

Step 1. The first thing to do is pick a quiet, comfortable, and tranquil place to sit, in a favorite chair or on the floor. Practice some deep breathing to get comfortable and focused.

Step 2. Next, go to a scene in your mind that is familiar and very calm, perhaps a scene that you recall from the beach, a movie you liked, or a favorite walk in the park that reminds you of complete tranquility. Make sure that the scene is clear, vivid, and detailed. Feel the scene and allow all of your senses to participate in the scene. Be sure to keep yourself completely comfortable physically as you bring in the sensory pleasures of the images of this scene. Spend about 2 to 3 minutes developing the scene: the smell, the touch, the feelings, and the sounds of the visual place. Be sure to envelop yourself in this comfortable and relaxed place.

Step 3. Now that you have a wonderful picture in your mind, freeze-frame it, lock it in, and then switch it off. Next, go back to your breathing and totally relaxed feeling in your chair or wherever you have placed yourself. Now, just breathe in and out with a blank screen in your mind. Do this for 2 minutes.

Step 4. Next, "flip the switch" and go back to that wonderful scene in your mental images. As you return to that relaxed and vivid place, pay attention to all the feelings and emotions associated with that scene. Spend 2 to 3 minutes with the scene. Now return to your breathing and a blank visual screen.

This procedure, Dr. Suinn's VMBR switching procedure, is quite simple and becomes nearly automatic with a bit of practice. Switching helps you learn to control the various elements of imagery. When you switch back and forth, you gain control of the imagery screen, taking command of the imagery and visualization process so that, over time, you can call up this technique at will. There is nothing magical about it. When you practice your golf game, you get better. When you practice your imagery, you get better pictures. When you put them both together—golf and imagery—the results are usually very positive.

TACKLE THE NEXT LEVEL

The next phase of the VMBR training is to take the imagery component one notch higher. Again, sit comfortably in your favorite chair or lie on the floor. Prepare yourself for deep breathing and full muscle relaxation.

Step 1. Switch on the relaxation scene described above. Now get tuned into that wonderful and relaxed place: the beach, the movie, the park—wherever you went in your mind's eye to relax fully. Go to that place and stay completely and fully with that tranquil scene. After 2 to 3 minutes, switch back to a blank screen, paying close attention to your breathing.

Enjoy the full body relaxation of breathing and relaxing with nothing on your mental picture screen.

Step 2. Now turn your attention to an athletic event: a swim race, a ski competition, a gymnastics meet, or a golf game, for example. Picture yourself as the participant, not the observer. Picture yourself winning, turning in a new personal record. Feel the emotion that sweeps over you as you cross the finish line, hear the cheers and people clapping, and touch and smell the sensations of winning and doing your best. Allow these images to be vivid and real; bring in all the kinesthetic sensations of winning the big one. Now that you have it in your mind, freeze-frame those winning emotions.

Step 3. Next, switch gears and get back to the relaxed frame. Remove the picture from your mind's eye and go back to your relaxed and effortless breathing. Do your deep, undisturbed breathing for 2 to 3 minutes. Now hit the switch and turn on that wonderful competitive winning scene. See the finish line; feel the tape, the water or the snow; soak up the emotions of letting down now that you have won the big race. Picture yourself as vividly as possible, letting your images be completely lucid. You can practice this on-and-off switching technique, increasing the amount of time that you spend in the imagery during each sequence. Twenty to 30 minutes a day of practice would be preferable. After all, practice makes perfect.

The VMBR technique can be used as frequently as you like. Most competitive athletes try to spend half an hour per day, 7 days a week, practicing this. In the survey of Olympic track and field athletes that I conducted with sports psychologist Jacqueline Golding, PhD, before the 1988 Olympics in Seoul, we found that some athletes practiced more frequently, and as the Olympics got closer, many practiced for several hours a day. It all depends on your particular style of preparation. Some athletes use VMBR only to deal with the stress of competition and reduce their anxiety levels when they visualize other athletes. Other competitors use VMBR to assist them with a challenging and icy giant slalom ski run or for any sport they compete in.

The applications are limitless. The important and operative word here is practice.

CHAPTER 9

Tap into the Power
of Dreams

You just woke up from a dream so vivid and detailed that you figure it
must mean something.

Is your subconscious sending you a message? Can your dreams affect
your actions in real life? Or can you manipulate your dreams as a sort of
nighttime mental practice?

Before the 1988 Olympic Marathon Trials, marathoner Margaret
Groos dreamed about them. "It was such an overwhelmingly positive
dream," she said. "I went through the whole thing, the whole race, the
whole strategy in my dream, and I won. I made the team, and the whole
elation of making the team and telling everyone . . . was very detailed and
vivid and specific. When I woke up, I had a very, very, positive feeling that
I was going to win."

The rest is history: Groos did in fact win the trials and qualify for the
Olympics.

After Jacqueline Golding, PhD, and I published our survey of elite athletes, which included results of survey questions about dreams and their
possible effects, we got phone calls from all over the country asking us for
more information about dreams—literature, data, anything. Researchers
and athletes alike were hungry to learn more about competitors' dreams.

The bad news was that there wasn't much in the libraries or computer databases, and we had to dig to unearth studies in this fascinating area. To date, there are only a handful of studies that have investigated athletes' dreams.

The questions that many people ask—and the ones we wanted answers to as well—are these.

- Is there a relationship between the amount of dreaming and performance levels?

- Does dreaming about success translate into higher performance levels?

- Do dream patterns change before upcoming competition?

- How do athletes view themselves in their dreams?

THE MUSINGS OF A MIND AT REST

Mental practice, as I explained earlier, is quite structured, but dreams and daydreams are much less rational. Dreams are often distorted, have crazy and bizarre streams of consciousness, and may symbolize other things. Some experts suggest that dreams might offer some keen insights about the psyche of competitive athletes. Dreaming of a successful performance may function as a kind of mental practice conducted on another, unconscious level.

The ancient Egyptians, Greeks, Romans, and Hebrews believed that dreams told us what would happen in the future. Sigmund Freud, MD, however, believed that dreams depict what we wish would happen—often wishes that are unacceptable during our daily lives. His book, *The Interpretation of Dreams*, expressed his belief that all dreams were tied to sexuality and unfinished business.

A disciple of Dr. Freud, Alfred Adler, MD, disagreed with his colleague's emphasis on the sexual meanings of dreams and the idea that dreams represent our wishes. He believed that the most important thing about dreams is the emotions they evoke in the dreamer—emotions that motivate the dreamer to act in waking life. For an athlete, for instance, feelings of joy and confidence in dreams might lead to better results in practice and competition. A minor study from two researchers from Pennsylvania State University in University Park lends support to this theory. The researchers interviewed 12 male gymnasts, seven of whom were selected for the 1976 US Olympic Team. These psychologists found that the athletes with the most vivid and frequent dreams had the best success in their events and were more likely to make the Olympic team than their teammates who dreamed less often.

PROBLEM SOLVING WHILE YOU SLEEP

Inventors, scientists, and writers have credited major accomplishments to ideas that came to them in dreams. In fact, dreams can help us when we are trying to resolve issues. Many of us have woken from a fitful sleep with some recollection of a dream sequence that may have led to something constructive.

Athletes often comment that they have dreams of winning, showing how they could be more successful in their quest for athletic excellence. Kim Jones, one of the best marathoners in the world, often dreams of victory. As of this writing, Kim has come in second at the Boston Marathon twice—although her dreams, in fact, are not of finishing second but of finishing with her hands high in the air, hitting the tape, as number one.

Some elite competitors claim that dreams alleviate stress. This might occur as athletes work out the stress of training and competing during their nighttime dream sessions. This relationship between dreams and waking mental practice definitely needs more attention, but one thing almost certainly holds true about dreams. Like mental imagery, practice makes perfect, if one is practicing—or dreaming of—the correct response. Practice makes imperfect, if one is practicing—or dreaming of—the wrong response. Dreaming of a successful performance may function as a kind of mental practice conducted on another, unconscious level.

If there is a connection between dream states and mentally rehearsing an event, then people who are vivid dreamers may have an edge on all of us. Connie Price-Smith, a shot and discus Olympian, told me just before the 1988 Seoul Olympics that she occasionally has a track dream. "In my dreams I always see the other competitors," she says. "If I can see the athletes in advance, then I certainly will be better prepared for the heat of competition."

Dreams have often been thought to have a problem-solving function, and, from this perspective, dreams of great athletic performances may show the dreamer new ways to train and compete successfully.

Some researchers claim that dreaming is all about memory and enhancing events from the day before. If this is true, then competitive athletes would be on active duty 24 hours a day—practicing during the day and then rehearsing workouts through their dream memories at night.

Margaret Groos has a unique way of dealing with positive and negative dreams. "I would say that there's obviously something wrong when I have disturbing dreams," she says. "The negative dreams that I have are typically during a negative phase in my training. This probably means that I didn't have confidence in my training for that week. It's very important to pay attention to these cues and change your training around so that you feel confident.

"These issues are important in setting up the proper type of workouts and avoidance of overtraining and injury. Building a winning attitude during workouts, where you feel like you've accomplished something, will help you refocus and assist in returning you to healthier dreams."

WEAVING YOUR OWN DREAMS

Lucid dreaming is a dream state where people are consciously aware that they are dreaming while they're dreaming. This may sound loony—except to those of you who may have experienced it—but there is strong scientific evidence for this notion. While in lucid dreaming, dreamers can intentionally control the events of their dreams. Researchers in a sophisticated dream lab at Stanford University have demonstrated that dreamers can actually signal their thoughts while still asleep, using prearranged signals such as eye movements and changes in breathing patterns to notify the research team.

When I originally published this book, scientists had begun to observe body movements during lucid dreams, suggesting neural pathways involved in motor skills are stimulated during dreams. Since then, research out of Germany suggests how lucid dreaming might play a key role in preparing athletes for competition. It appears that, if an athlete has already learned a certain sensory-motor skill with some proficiency, lucid dreaming can help that athlete master the skill. Repeated movements in particular—throwing a baseball, for instance, or rapid slalom movements on snow skis, skateboards, and snowboards—can be substantially improved during lucid dreaming.

WHAT YOU SEE WHEN YOU WAKE UP

When Dr. Golding and I conducted our survey of Olympians, we asked them a number of questions about their dream activity, both during the day and at night. Here is a snapshot of what they told us.

- More than ⅘ dreamed about their sports, and the same number dreamed about competition.

- Women tended to report or remember their dreams more often.

- The athletes who trained the hardest also reported the most dream activity and perhaps the clearest recall.

- Athletes who reported high levels of commitment to making the Olympic team and those who had made the most stressful sacrifices to prepare for the trials dreamed more frequently of participating and competing.

- Athletes who worked with a coach also dreamed more frequently of competition.

- Nearly half of our sample reported dreams of successful outcomes. Athletes who were younger, less educated, or unmarried reported more frequent success in their dream competitions.

- Field athletes, such as pole vaulters and high jumpers, reported the most frequent success in dreams, and marathoners reported the least. (Field athletes, according to our earlier studies, also do more mental practice than other athletes.)

- Older athletes between ages 29 and 45 and those most committed to making the team were frequent daydreamers.

- Nearly one-third of the athletes reported successful daydreams "always" or "almost always." Half chose one of these top two frequency categories.

- Athletes who were the most committed to making the Olympic team were more likely to report successful daydreams.

Our findings suggest that age and education and whether the athletes participated in track, field, or marathon do have some influence on whether the athletes dream of successful outcomes. Beyond that, however, commitment to making the team and the intense sacrifice of getting there is the best predictor of success in dreams.

In 1989, Dr. Golding and I, along with psychologist and sports consultant Kay Porter, PhD, studied 210 athletes from the 1984 National Masters Track and Field Championship and 446 from the 1987 Championship. Here's what we found.

- Half the athletes reported dreaming about competition—usually about winning.

- Younger athletes and those who practiced visualization were the most likely to dream about competition.

- Athletes who dreamed about competition tended to be more anxious.

- Those who dreamed of success reported less depression in their lives.

- Some athletes who dreamed of their sports reported personal bests during the competition.

NIGHTTIME PREDICTIONS
OF DAYTIME SUCCESS

As you can see, athletes, especially Olympians, seem to dream frequently. One group of track and field Olympians told us that they dreamed of competition every night. Most dreamed about competition and could specifically recall certain dream events on a regular basis. It seems reasonable that athletes who remember dreams more frequently and vividly in general are more likely to remember dreams about athletic competitions.

Danny Everett, 1988 Olympic sprinting gold medalist who set a world record in the 400 meters, explains that he often has problems with sleep, but these apparently don't affect his success as a world-class sprinter. "Right before the finals of the 400 meters in Seoul, I didn't sleep well," he said. "I don't remember dreaming of a race or of a winning experience. I dreamed more of my preparation and training for the race. I seem to place more value on hard work and thorough training than just winning a race . . . maybe that's why it shows up in my dreams as just preparing to race."

In our research with Olympians, we found that many athletes dreamed of both practice and competition. In fact, the competitors who trained the most hours daily were the ones who apparently carried their desire to succeed and work ethic into their dreams with them. These athletes have a strong commitment to making the Olympic team. Perhaps dreaming is more prolific among these dedicated, intense athletes because they put in many grueling hours and make major sacrifices to make their dream of qualifying for the Olympics come true. This type of all-or-nothing commitment to being an Olympic athlete would certainly preoccupy one's waking and sleeping hours. These athletes eat, sleep, and breathe their sports in a literal sense; they sleep it by dreaming about it.

The great news about dreams is that they may lend a helping hand to mental practice and skill development in any sport. The bad news is that scientists have not studied this topic very thoroughly. It seems clear, however, that in some cases, waking performance is directly related to dream performance.

The relation can be a positive one or a negative one. Groos told me of some dreams with unhappy outcomes. "I've also dreamed that I've done badly in a race, and then I do," she said. "They always come true—the power of both the positive and the negative. In 1984, I dreamed the night before the Olympic Trials that I finished fifth. . . . I woke up that morning and told my friend that I was rooming with that I had a dream that I finished fifth. She said not to worry about the dream, that I'd make the Olympic team." And what happened? Groos finished fifth and failed to qualify for the Olympics. Four years later in 1988, she shifted gears and focused more on the positive and did qualify for the Olympic team.

Dreams are deeply personal and usually highlight very emotional events. Jeff Atkinson, 1988 Olympic gold medalist in the 1500 meters, told me, "My dreams don't really focus on winning . . . they are more feeling-oriented. I dream more in emotions than pictures. These feelings could be a big win or even a big loss. Sometimes I wake with a feeling of tremendous success. And I have this really supreme feeling all over!" Clearly, we need to pursue more study in this fascinating area of the dream lives of athletes. The idea of dreams as a form of mental practice is very appealing.

Atkinson and other great athletes make us wonder about the power of dreams. His dreams suggest a nighttime mental practice session. They also suggest a means of improving mental toughness, an ability to control one's emotional behavior, and a way to cope with the stress of competition. Anyway you cut it, dreams offer wonderful insights into our deeper selves.

CHAPTER 10

Get Psyched without Losing Your Edge

Precompetition preparation is all about getting ready physically as well as psychologically. Most elite athletes will tell you that they're confident that physically, they're well prepared, but they often worry that they haven't covered their bases in the emotional and psychological areas.

Mark Plaatjes, the marathon gold medalist at the 1993 Track and Field World Championship in Stuttgart, Germany, had trained extensively for his marathon quest. He even memorized the contours and hills of the marathon course from maps and pictures that he had received from friends. And yet he continued to worry about certain stages of the race and other competitors. He may have come close to being overprepared and allowing all the details of the 26.2-mile race to seep into his mind and cause him many sleepless nights.

So how do you get psyched and, more important, not get overpsyched? Breathing, meditation, imagery, and visualization, explained in earlier chapters, are all very important strategies when learning how to stay tuned up without getting too aroused. But when it comes to the day of competition, what are the other things that you can do to prepare emotionally?

DISTRACTIONS CAN DESTROY CONCENTRATION

Little things such as travel, getting equipment and clothing to the competition site, and arranging for lodging and food are important and need to be organized well in advance. The mental side of precompetition arrangements includes a final emotional tune-up with breathing exercises, a review of the goals you have set in advance, and a full mental and visual rehearsal of the game plan. It's important at this point to passively clear the mind. This means not forcing yourself to clear your mind. Let go, close your eyes, and get ready to move to the next phase of preparing for competition. But don't force it or let yourself feel rushed.

Coaches often will ask athletes not to talk to the press or spectators so that they don't incur any psychological distractions. Athletes at this stage of readiness need to focus on the competition, and socializing and hanging out with the media and friends can come later.

CONTROL IS CRUCIAL

The important thing to remember about keeping your edge is to be in control. You, the athlete, must know and feel that you are in control. You should feel so confident that you can expect the unexpected. You should have considered things like weather (including excessive heat and humidity), crowd noise, unfamiliar surroundings, food, sleep, and daily routines well in advance. After a long overseas flight, you need to anticipate the effects of jet lag. Before the 1988 Seoul Games, the United States Olympic Committee sent out guidelines suggesting that competitors arrive at the Games one day in advance for each hour of time zone that was passed. So, for example, all the West Coast athletes should have gone to South Korea 16 days in advance to cope effectively with the physiological drag of jet lag.

By this time, you would have anticipated food and cultural differences (if you were competing in a different country) and that you might not be sleeping through the night. At the Los Angeles Olympics in 1984, the dorms at UCLA where the athletes were housed were extremely noisy. Many coaches made prior arrangements to move some athletes to hotel rooms 24 hours before competition. At the Barcelona Olympics in 1992, there were high levels of heat and humidity and little air-conditioning. Many athletes were sleep-deprived and quite uncomfortable, but they had anticipated these problems, so they were less disconcerted than would be expected. Such issues must be discussed and dealt with many months in advance. Nancy Ditz, 1988 Olympic marathoner, has always had a hard time with heat. So she goes out of her way not only to train in heat but also to visualize the emotions that might accompany a warm day on the marathon course. You, too, should make the necessary adjustments before an event.

Even for developing athletes who have yet to taste international competition, it is still important to plan ahead. My younger daughter, who was a competitive gymnast at the National Academy of Artistic Gymnastics, competed all over the Northwest at 15 different gyms throughout the competitive season. She and her teammates often complained that when they got to a gym, they found that the uneven bars were old and not in good shape. The floor exercise mat was not up to standard and didn't allow for good punch and rotation on tumbling passes. Worst of all, she reported that many gyms were so small that she could not get a solid run on the vault. These are all issues that her coach should have briefed the team about well in advance. A picture of the gym, a brief description of their equipment, and a discussion of what to expect before the meet would have alleviated some of the distress when the athletes arrived at the competition venue. If you're a coach, it's never too early to start preparing your athletes for the unexpected.

FINISHING TOUCHES

As competition day nears, it is important for athlete and coach to assess skill level, analyze the game plan one last time, and then put all of their collective energies into focus. It is now time to stop analyzing and focus on integrating all the mental training strategies that the athlete has learned. Remember: Overanalysis leads to paralysis.

Don't think about correcting technique at this point; instead, go with the skills that you have been working on for many months. This is the time to use all the breathing, imagery, and mental rehearsal strategies and integrate them with the physical game plan. This is not the time to introduce a last-minute mental focus plan. Some coaches might try too hard and introduce a mantra or tune-up strategy just before competition day. This can be a terrible distraction that ends up confusing the athlete. Stick with the game plan, follow through with the mental preparation that you have worked on, stay focused, and keep your edge.

In our survey of 1,200 elite athletes that I mentioned earlier, we found, for example, that during the summer just before the September 1988 Games, the athletes who qualified for the Olympic team trained more and had more mental practice than those who didn't make the team. We felt that for some Olympians, a final tune-up was a good idea, but for others who were introduced to new imagery and visualization training for the first time, this might have been counterproductive. For this reason, an imagery audiotape that you or your coach has made is a very useful tool to carry with you from the training regimen to the day of final competition. It is always with you, it is familiar, and you can play the imagery tape as many times as you like in preparation for your event. It is a convenient way to reorient yourself and stay in a familiar emotional setting—even though you might be hundreds or thousands of miles from home.

THE BIG DAY

On competition day, it doesn't matter if you are a beginning jogger running your first 5-K, a college diving athlete going for the NCAA title, or a figure skater competing for a spot on the US Olympic team. Competition is competition. It is an exciting time and you're full of energy. How you use that energy is usually what decides the outcome of the event. Review your goals for that competition, both on paper and in your mind, and keep reminding yourself to stay with your game plan. Eliminate distractions or any event that might promote negativity. Again, avoid the media. This is not a time to be interviewed or put under the klieg lights. That will come later.

When you get to the actual site of competition, whether it's a gym, track, ice rink, or ski course, check out your surroundings. Notice the obvious: the weather, temperature and humidity, physical surroundings such as viewing area and bleachers, officials, spectators, cameras and media personnel, and unfamiliar faces. Check out all the sights and sounds to see if they fit your preconceived notion of what you expected. If they do, fine; if they seem different, this is also fine. Remember, you have visualized this place before, and you have also learned to expect the unexpected. This is all part of your precompetition tune-up and mental preparation.

LAST-MINUTE ADJUSTMENTS

Next, it is time to consider any last changes or adjustments that you want to make before your competition. There should be very few modifications, because you have rehearsed this day thoroughly. At times, however, there might be a quick or minor adjustment made to a strategy. Survey the participants and note who is there, who is competing, and who are the ones that you will be aiming to beat. Again, there should be no surprises, because in your mind's eye, you have traveled here before and seen all of these athletes months in advance.

Now it is time to move toward your "perfect timing and energy zone"—what I call the PTEZ period—usually just 30 minutes before the event. The PTEZ simply means that you are ready, and you are stepping up to that next level of fine-tuning. You are reaching for the optimal level of positive energy and positive arousal. All the jitters and butterflies are there, but you are now taking control of this anxiety and converting it to positive and productive competition energy in anticipation of a great event.

Some athletes use breathing, meditation, and arousal or stress reduction techniques at this point. Other athletes go in the other direction and move toward more arousal and stimulation to increase energy levels. Remember (and this is especially important for coaches), every athlete is different, has different emotional needs, and responds differently to the precompetition tune-up. Some athletes need more energy just before competition; some need less. Know these limits within yourself and practice setting these limits, recording them in a diary and getting comfortable with the perfect timing and energy zone. This is a critical period, and each athlete needs special attention.

RITUALS FOR READINESS

Often athletes have pregame rituals or idiosyncrasies that allow them to get into the PTEZ. I mentioned previously that former NBA all-star Patrick Ewing secludes himself with a personal stereo and some special music. Other athletes like to just walk around talking to themselves, scribble notes on a pad, call a spouse or loved one, or just sit with their eyes closed in the corner of a room. Some athletes just sit quietly and indulge themselves in a John Grisham thriller. My oldest daughter, Shoshana, would always wear two pairs of socks (usually her MJ-23 ones) right before her competitions. She would roll them a certain way, tuck them, and make sure they fit properly. I'm not sure this is the precise reason she made it to the state tennis championships, but I know that certain rituals do help an athlete get focused and centered.

Whatever the ritual, coaches need to honor and respect it. Teammates need to be sensitive to individual and team rituals and allow fellow athletes to have their own unique experiences before competition. My younger daughter loved to pack at least two teddy bears for her gymnastic competitions; then, at the last minute, she would choose one from her bag and give it a big hug before she competed. Superstar basketball player Michael Jordan noted in his book *Air Time* that when he took the floor for warmups as a Chicago Bull, he would always search the stadium seats for the loving and supportive smile of his dad, James. He said that after he located his dad in the bleachers, he knew his game was going to be solid.

By having a ritual, a superstition, or an idiosyncratic warmup routine, athletes take control of their environments and filter out any negative distractions that might interfere with the pending competition. For those athletes and coaches who have never developed a PTEZ ritual, here are some basics to consider.

1. Begin with some breathing exercises.

2. Next do a short imagery and visualization session. This should be done with familiar scenes and images from prior successful events.

3. Use positive self-talk and positive affirmations to help yourself get ready. Remind yourself that you have been here before, you are very fit, you're ready to go, and you feel at the top of your game.

4. Finally, remind yourself of your personal mantra or saying that is the cue for you to do your best. Some athletes like "in the flow" or "in the zone" to remind them that they are truly in the PTEZ.

Most of all, remember that you are there to compete, do your very best, and enjoy yourself. Peter Jacobsen, one of the most successful golf touring pros over the past 26 years, recently told me: "Above all, you have to go out there and have fun. If you don't build in that component, it gets very stale, and you can burn out."

PART THREE

SPORT-SPECIFIC
MENTAL
PRACTICE

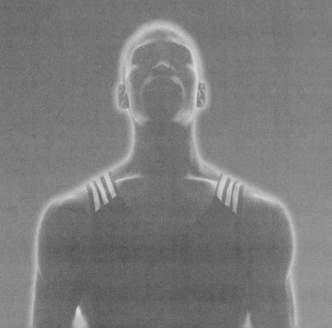

CHAPTER 11

Cycling: Improve Your Style and Power

The cycling athlete of today differs from those in the early 1980s, says Chris Carmichael, Lance Armstrong's personal coach for the past 13 years and a member of the 1984 Olympic Cycling Team. "We have kids coming into the sport who are better educated about physiology, kinesiology, and psychology," he told me. "They have trained and competed in other sports, so they're more sophisticated about training in general. They are better-quality and more versatile athletes. They come from football, basketball, skiing, and cross-country, so they know the demands of endurance and pain thresholds. In the old days, a cyclist was more of a fringe athlete who didn't really understand the nuances of the sport."

Cyclists are hardly fringe athletes these days. The top performers routinely break the million-dollar mark every year, and top US pro Lance Armstrong, arguably the best cyclist ever, reportedly earns between $17 million and $20 million a year. And those higher potential earnings draw more and more top athletes from other sports.

From a psychological standpoint, Carmichael, a former top racer himself, sees very different kinds of athletes coming through the US Olympic Training Center in Colorado Springs. He can tell immediately which athletes have the desire to win, the ability to handle endurance training and tolerate pain, and, most important, the capability to handle the distractions that are an inevitable part of competing.

"I think the most important aspect to the psyche of cyclists, both team and individual athletes, is how they cope with distractions," says Carmichael. "Whether it is pain, weather conditions, personality clashes, travel, or general politics of racing, the real champions are the ones who can get beyond the moment, put distractions on the back burner, and stay completely focused." Ultimately, he told me, "Cyclists are limited only by how much desire and discipline they bring to the sport."

MENTAL MASTERS

Chris Carmichael was a member of the 1984 Olympic Cycling Team, a member of five world-championship teams, and has been the exclusive coach for six-time Tour de France winner Lance Armstrong for the past 13 years.

Chris Witty competed in the 1998 Nagano winter Olympics and the 2002 Salt Lake City games as a speed skater. In between, she squeezed in the summer Sydney 2000 Olympics as a cyclist.

Chris Baldwin was the winner of the gold medal in the 2003 Pan Am Games in the 50-K time trial.

Jim Edmark, a former track runner, was the 1993 and 1996 Oregon District Criterium Champion and is sponsored by Finlandia.

Brad Gebhard competed in the 1988 Olympic Trials and has raced all over the world.

Mark Gorski was a member of the 1980 Olympic Team, a gold medalist in the 1984 Los Angeles Olympics in the matched sprint event, and a silver medalist in the 1987 Pan Am Games. He set a world record in the 200 meters and is presently managing the US Postal Service team.

DO YOUR HOMEWORK

While you can use mental practice strategies both before and after a race, you'll do much of your mental practice at home and during training rides. And mental practice can benefit recreational cyclists as well.

Survey your goals. The first step in mental training is to assess your own abilities and goals, says Carmichael. There are certain elements that you must be aware of to be a great cycling athlete, he says. Cyclists should:

- Determine and articulate their goals early in their training.

- Bring lofty dreams into a realistic focus.

Vaidila Kungys was the runner-up in the 1993 Junior National Criterium Championship and finished 39th at the World Championship in the 80-mile race in Perth, Australia.

Karl Maxon was the 1986 US National Champion and has secured more than 118 wins throughout his career. He raced the pro circuit for Team Sachs/Fila from 1991 to 1993 and raced on the Fagor French Pro Team in 1987.

Rebecca Twigg was a silver medalist in the 1984 Olympics in road racing; she followed in Barcelona at the 1992 games with a bronze in the Olympic pursuit; she is a three-time world record holder in the pursuit and a six-time world champion.

Leann Warren was a world-class middle-distance runner, US Olympian, and four-time NCAA Champion in the 800 and 1500 meters. She moved to cycling in 1992 because of injuries. In her second year of cycling competition, she won the Oregon District Criterium.

- Use short-term racing goals to act as benchmarks to assist training strategies.

And regardless of the event, whether you're road racing, riding in time trials, or sprinting in a velodrome, you must know your capabilities.

Stay tough. Cycling can require a lot of mental toughness, especially if you don't ride with a team, says 1984 Olympic cycling gold medalist Mark Gorski. "You have to find your own reason for being out there in the icy rain, fighting traffic, working that hard," he says. "The fans are not out there giving us strokes, and television has not relegated cycling to Sunday afternoon prime time, and people still question our sanity. There isn't a lot of emotional support for the sport."

See the victory. Rebecca Twigg, who stunned the cycling world by returning from retirement in time to grab a bronze medal at the 1992 Olympics, still loves training and competition after racing for 15 years. She says that any good cycling athlete does imagery and mental practice whether or not they're aware of it. She specifically and consciously imagined victory. "I used to imagine, what if I won and who would I thank when I had my gold medal dangling from my neck? I used to picture myself winning, standing high above at the podium. I would use that image to reinforce my confidence for my next race. In the Olympics, I carried with me a set of images from that precious moment, and those visuals usually enhanced the preparation for my next big race."

Study the course. According to 1993 and 1996 Oregon District Criterium Champion Jim Edmark, you need a strong visual sense of the race course before you get out there and race. "Unless I visualize myself from the racing perspective on the course around other cyclists, I will not have a competitive race," he says. Edmark notes that he has to see and feel the course before each race to get a good sense of the competition. He goes to each course well in advance and takes a comfortable ride through it so that he can mentally record the hills, the contours, the shoulder, and the scenery. All of this information gets stored in the "what" and "where" centers of his brain for a later date.

Mentally ride the route. You have to visualize yourself riding that specific race course, experiencing the whole course—the contours, the bumps, and the scenery, says pro racer and 1986 US National Champion Karl Maxon. "You have to see, hear, and feel your gear ratios for the entire

SECRETS OF SUCCESS:
CHRIS BALDWIN

Chris Baldwin was born in 1975 in Boulder, Colorado, a great place to train and become a champion in road racing. Indeed, he won a gold medal in the 2003 Pan Am Games in the 50-K time trial. In his first 3 years as a professional, Chris has won eight races.

But Baldwin's success hasn't been simple luck. Like any athlete, he's had to overcome injury and failure.

"My most difficult aspect of athletics are setbacks," he says. "They are tough, and I have to know that they will help me in the long run; they build my character."

Baldwin copes by staying logical and figuring out the most efficient ways to get over setbacks.

"When I had my knee surgery [in 2001], I had to find other ways to succeed by turning to weight training when I couldn't ride," he told me recently.

Baldwin has several suggestions for staying focused, including:

- Stay in the moment. (Baldwin uses a mantra of "Now, now, now.")

- Expect ups and downs while you're racing. Stay even keeled.

- Attack your faults. ("I suffer more than others in heat and humidity, so I prepare for it," he says.)

- Keep a comprehensive training journal, and set short-term and long-term goals.

- Get up and out the door at the same time every day.

- Always keep in mind the end result: getting on the podium.

course, imaging the smooth and rough parts throughout." This is visual rehearsal.

Know the other competitors. Vaidila Kungys, runner-up in the 1993 Junior National Criterium Championship, often asks to see race sign-up sheets before the start of his events so that he'll know who the other competitors are. He wants to visualize all the competitors and prepare for their tactics on the course. "I visualize certain athletes who climb poorly, so that is when I will make a move," he explains. "I visualize some cyclists who are just great competitors. I watch certain people and learn techniques from them. I value the great ones because, like any sport, if you watch carefully, you can learn a lot. The imagery gets locked in when you see the best in the field."

"See" the other guy. Rebecca Twigg usually visualizes her competitor, especially in the one-on-one pursuit, when two cyclists begin at opposite sides of the track. "I always think about a particular athlete, especially someone whom I don't usually beat," she says. Brad Gebhard, who competed in the 1988 Olympic Trials and has raced all over the world, also concentrates on visualizing the competition. "I need to know who is out there and what their strengths are. So my preparatory images deal with other athletes and what they are capable of doing on the course. I have to know each person's strengths and capabilities in order to gauge their power in the sprint."

Time your visualization right. Edmark does his race visualization shortly before the big event. "I never do too much visualization weeks in advance," he says. "My strategy is to stay calm and relaxed with lots of deep breathing so I don't get too revved up before a big competition. Then, about 2 days before my big races, I go into a deep visualization strategy where I see and feel lots of different aspects of the race. I picture myself at different points on the course, I see myself in a pack of cyclists, I feel the burning in my thighs as I climb, and I see the scenery, the trees and brush, the guardrails. I take in those external environmental cues, and I am also keenly aware of my place in the pack and my energy level."

Watch yourself win. Visualization for Edmark is about seeing himself at the head of the pack, seeing other riders tire and fade into the background, and making his surge. He sees the big gap open up and then himself crossing the finish line, finishing with lots of energy while guys behind him are looking tired and spent. Edmark never consciously sits and listens to his internal thoughts or waits for images to appear. They just do. "Every workout I do, especially on hills or over some rough terrain, I find myself automatically seeing and hearing the sounds of a major cycling event," Edmark says. "I constantly see myself in the pack, breaking away and then winning. I often throw my hands up in the air just like the guys at the Tour de

```
SECRETS OF SUCCESS:
REBECCA TWIGG
```

Showing 'em How It's Done

To stay tuned up, Olympic champion Rebecca Twigg does a lot of training year-round. Her racing season is from March to October, but she rides all the time, doing endurance and speed work. She listens to her favorite music on long rides and trains at altitude in Flagstaff, Arizona, a refreshing difference from sea level. For cross-training, she jogs, uses weights, skis, and does indoor riding on a turbo trainer.

France as they cross the finish line; I can even hear the roar of the crowd. It is all part of my daily mental training."

Talk to yourself. Kungys also uses a mantra or verbal chant when he trains: "Looking good, feeling strong, nothing can go wrong!" He uses this often to remind himself cognitively that he is tough and ready to compete, and you can use such a mantra during the race itself as well. This is an example of self-talk that works for cyclists.

PUT ON YOUR GAME FACE

Former track star Leann Warren, who switched to cycling in 1992, notes that runners often have a hard time transitioning from foot races to cycling events. "Cycling is psychologically very different," she says. "If you go out hard in a cycling race (a common strategy for middle-distance track runners), you'll get eaten alive. Athletes will just draft off you. That's not the same outcome in track running. It can be very frustrating when you first learn the sport."

These tips can help you hone your head game.

Be prepared for variables. Warren brought a strong physiological base to the sport of cycling but still has many doubts about her abilities. "In track, I had such wonderful confidence," she says. "I just went out there and ran my race, at my pace, at my comfort level, and usually won. In cycling, I haven't attained that confidence base yet. The strategy is so radically different that I don't really know myself with this sport. Even in my visualization work, the imagery was so much clearer in track because of the confidence I brought to the sport. I could easily visualize my pace, my kick, and my win. In cycling, there are so many other variables to throw you off. Cyclists are so aggressive, so very tactical; the pace and the pack are very deceptive forces. You have to be prepared in your mind and body for a sudden shift in energy, force, and sprints." This is the kind of thinking that the winners use to focus and deal with distractions.

Stay tuned to hazards. Competitive cycling is a balance between safety and risk taking—knowing when to make a move that will be safe, energy-efficient, and effective. Even as you monitor yourself internally, checking your breathing and fatigue level, you also have to be mindful of cars, other bikes, obstacles in the road, and other distractions. The slightest touch of tires can cause a serious crash, for instance. Racers such as Twigg and Chris Witty constantly catalog in their internal files all the hazards along the road so that they can spend most of their time focused on the race.

Ration your energy. Cycling is about riding intelligently, according to the experts. You have to start with deep, full breathing and know that your energy level will change over a period of 4 hours. You have to conserve energy and know when to expend it. You have to know when to break away and whether you will have to expend that kind of energy many times in a race. Do I go now or do I wait for another opportunity? You have to know the pace, the strategy, and when to stay calm and when to surge. If you surge now, it is one less surge in your energy bank account to write checks on in the future. This is a perfect example of how breathing helps calm the mind and muscles for the challenges of a cycling surge.

Watch the other guy. When Edmark sees fatigue in another competitor, he makes his move. He watches for poor pedal strokes or the bobbing up and down of an athlete's back that signals him it's time to surge. "When I see that other racers are struggling, I know it is time for my attack phase, and I will surge at this point and move to another energy level."

Patience is key. Warren emphasizes that racing is all about patience and knowing when to surge and break away from the pack. "In cycling, there is a lot of variance in your methods. One minute you can be chitchatting away, and the next minute you can be in complete oxygen debt. A few seconds later, you can be relaxing and enjoying the scenery. It is one extreme or the other."

React quickly. Gebhard has had much mental training, perhaps more than most elite or Olympic athletes. He spent five consecutive winters at the US Olympic Committee Center in Colorado Springs working with an assortment of sport psychologists and other professionals. "You know, in theory, this imagery business works great," he says, "but when you get right down to the race, the best athlete is the one who is best prepared to deal with any difficult situation. You need to be able to react quickly and with confidence in those tight spots." That's where experience comes in. The more you consciously integrate mind and body techniques, the better it all clicks.

BE READY FOR PAIN

Edmark is also a former track runner and knows the feelings and emotions of being in tight places. He was a 31:20 10-K racer and knows about energy conservation, positioning, and the ever-important surge and final kick. He learned a lot from his track days, such as knowing when to make a move based on the emotions of his competitors. "When I am racing in a criterium race, I have to not only listen to my pace and my fatigue level, but also be mindful of the other racers," he explains. "I have to anticipate the pain. The trick is to know how to deal effectively with it. When you reach that threshold of discomfort, you need to convert it to positive energy, positive thoughts, and positive overdrive."

Edmark practices visualization strategies but also does much kinesthetic imagery, concentrating on how he feels rather than what he sees or hears or what his mood is. He constructs imagery around being fluid, effortless, and very efficient as he races. He feels the race and has all his senses tune in to the pain and inevitable discomfort. During a mental practice session, he gets himself into a psychological framework that activates the energy from a race to the point of feeling fatigue and pain—lots of pain. When the pain comes on, he converts that sensation to aggression, telling himself that he has to stay tough and not give in to the pain. "It's funny, but my best races have been when I didn't feel any pain. It's always there, but I guess I converted it very effectively both in my mental practice and then in the competition." This conversion process allows him to go to that next level of competition, which uses one form of energy and redefines it as aggressiveness.

SECRETS OF SUCCESS: KARL MAXON

Tips from a Cycling Champ

Karl Maxon joined the cycling scene soon after he ran a 2:47 marathon at age 16 and then was injured. He wanted to train hard, and running was too tough on his body. In his first bicycle race, he won a $360 Univega Grand Rally touring bike—and got completely hooked on cycling.

Retired from cycling now, Maxon is intense about his new career, being a certified public accountant with a Big Eight firm. Maxon looks intense whether he's discussing riding through the Italian Alps or studying accounting procedures. "When I used to ride, I would ride to burn fat, train for hills, practice my gearing, do intervals, and rehearse pedal technique. Everything has a purpose."

First and foremost, says Maxon, you must have base endurance. That means solid hours of training to develop a base level of fitness. Next you must have an excellent anaerobic threshold that will lead to pure horsepower. He considers churning a gear ratio of 53/15 at 23 miles per hour on the flats for 4 to 5 hours a great way to get that pure horsepower. Anaerobic threshold refers to the point at which your oxygen supply can't produce the energy you need. Raising your anaerobic threshold will improve your endurance, helping you exercise longer and faster. He also suggests doing 30- to 45-second intervals on hills in a 39/19 gear ratio so that you can get your heartbeat up to maximum capacity.

Here is Maxon's seven-step prescription for great racing.

1. Trust what you do.

2. Don't let people undermine your confidence.

3. Have total belief in your training regimens.

4. Believe in your coach and trainer.

5. Train without a coach if you want, as long as you set your goals and have a written training schedule.

6. Study physiology; know the body.

7. Set your goals high, maintain confidence, and train hard.

"It is an attitude. I see so many cyclists who give in to the pain. Their faces show the fatigue, and then they give up," he says. "I know that place, I have been there myself, and I know when it is about to hit me. I prepare mentally for that moment in the race; I seize that moment, convert it, and feel a new positive attitude."

Gebhard is a firm believer in training physically tough. He says there's a direct relationship between training physically and emotionally. Gebhard has raced all over the world, including 3 weeks of intensive training and racing on the island of Guadeloupe in the Caribbean. "The roads are bumpy and very erratic down there," he points out. Getting used to tough physical conditions can help you tough it out mentally during your next event.

HOW TO DEAL WITH SETBACKS

Kungys lives and trains on the West Coast. He is convinced that to race strongly, you have to be mentally prepared for each race. He says that you must visualize everything and anything that can happen, good or bad, during a race. "I want to expect the unexpected and be prepared for any event during a 5-hour race," he says. "I actually visualize crashes during my preparation. Not that it's pleasant to see myself wipe out on cold, hard cement, but I need to prepare for the extreme worst situation. I see myself racing hard, the number two cyclist crashes, and the next three go down in a tangled mess of bikes and bruised legs. It is not a pretty sight. But then I realize that I'm not hurt. I get up, briskly reminding myself that I am still competing and very much in the race. I check my bike and make sure it is still okay to ride, and then my last sequence of imagery is racing back to the pack of cyclists."

These tips will help you deal with whatever occurs while cycling.

Channel your rage. "Cycling is about staying in top physical shape, but also being mentally prepared," says former racer Guard Wells. Once, when he crashed during a big race, Wells found himself on the ground, shaken but not hurt—and enraged that the accident had knocked him out of the pack. "I found myself reacting physically and emotionally to the anger," he says. "As soon as I got myself together, I visualized bridging back to the pack, clearing the pack, and winning the race. The visuals were so vivid; perhaps it was a reaction to the anger that strengthened the imagery process." His mental images helped him overcome his accident and finish strongly.

This vignette is not dissimilar to the astonishing crash and strong recovery by Lance Armstrong in his July 2003 victory at his fifth Tour de France race.

Visualize weather conditions. Like track, cycling has a strong mental preparation component. Much prerace preparation must take place in your visualization training. Warren suggests, for example, that you rehearse for any weather condition, racing in wind and rain as well as riding on a very hot, humid day.

Remember your goals. Cycling can be a lonely sport. "You train for hours at a time by yourself," says Kungys. "It is windy, cold, dark, and sometime dangerous. Drivers in some places have no respect for cycling athletes. So you have to remember your goals, your purpose, and your reason for training so diligently. Remember to check in with those objectives whenever you feel you need to."

Imagine dealing with illness. It's important to take yourself through events such as crashes and bad weather so you know how to handle any athletic trauma, says Kungys. "I also imagine myself not feeling well—weak or sick or congested—so that I can anticipate that outcome as well," he says. "I let myself have a few minutes of feeling rotten, then I shift the imagery screen to feeling stronger and healthier. Then I notch it up to feeling absolutely great."

COPING WITH INJURY

Warren came to cycling with many credentials. She was a world-class middle-distance runner and US Olympian but also knew a lot about her body and its vulnerabilities. "I really went through a tough time moving from track running and road racing to being a competitive cyclist," she says. "I have a sense of loss and grief over not being able to completely fulfill my goals as a runner. It's hard to replace that special energy and acknowledgment from my track days. But after nine knee surgeries, it was time to hang up the spikes and refocus my energies to cycling. I needed to find other ways to gain approval and personal fulfillment."

As with any sport, coping with an injury-induced layoff from cycling takes a certain amount of mental rehab to help you get back in the saddle, mentally and physically. And injuries do happen. Here, Warren and two other noted cyclists share how they used mental strategies to deal with injury-related setbacks to training and racing.

Prepare for injury. Warren is still grieving over the loss of her almost-perfect track career. No doubt she would have been an Olympic medalist and road runner for years to come. But injury caused her to carve out a new path—a perfect spokesperson for how attitude adjustment can help cyclists mentally recover from injury and disappointment. Here's her advice on minimizing the psychological impact of injury.

- Assume that you are going to get injured, perhaps many times, in your career. Expect it. Plan for it psychologically.

- Know that when you are injured, you need time to recover physically and emotionally. Try to see the big picture—that sport is part of the continuum of life, and you will recover if you allow yourself healing time.

- Have enough confidence to say, "I'm okay." Let go of obsessive-compulsive training patterns and take more time off for active and passive rest.

- Know that with or without sport, you are a good, solid, confident person. Your entire identity and self-esteem should not be tied to a sport.

Finally, says Warren, go easy on yourself. Healing and getting back into shape can be tough.

Keep mind and body active. World-class racer Gebhard had to overcome a broken collarbone, chipped patella, broken back, and a host of other injuries that knocked him out of racing for a while. "My knee surgery kept me in a full leg cast for 4 months, and I got severely depressed," he says. "My leg started to atrophy, and I thought I would never get back to the sport." He lost much of his confidence in himself and his body. During his rehabilitation period, Gebhard worked on his body but concentrated on his emotional state as well. "It got so bad at one point that I started riding with my full leg cast on, pedaling around town, just to build up my confidence. Doing mental imagery during rehab is good for the body but really good for the soul. It puts you back into the action and prepares you for your comeback. I also used a lot of creative diversion while I was sick; I read, I studied, and I had more of a social life. I channeled that compulsive energy into some other aspects of my life. It was a healthy distraction."

Prevent burnout with downtime. Kungys is a true believer in downtime—active rest away from the sport of cycling—because of the mental and physical fatigue factor. "I read, practice guitar, and shoot baskets just to get out of the routine," he says. "I often have so much anxiety before a race that I have to get away from the tension. I distract myself whenever I can, knowing that I have trained well and now need to just relax and not over-amp before the big race."

THE ROLE OF THE COACH

The US Cycling Federation spends most of its time training coaches in mental practice, goal setting, and team-building methods, points out Carmichael. This is an important issue that has caused a raging debate in the United States among many national governing bodies for various sports, as some people believe that coaches need only be able to teach physical skills specific to each sport. "We feel that cycling coaches are valued human beings," explains Carmichael. "They are not just there to hold hands in a crisis. These are talented, well-trained, professional people who deserve our admiration and respect. If we don't train them in all aspects of the sport, including state-of-the-art mental practice and visualization strategies, we are doing the whole sport a disservice. Cycling athletes have a special intimate relationship with their coaches, so everyone needs to be in the training loop."

Aside from formal mental work, coaches should also play a role in helping athletes relax when their work is through, Carmichael has noted. After coaching Lance Armstrong to his sixth Tour de France victory, Carmichael focused primarily not on planning for the future, but on celebrating.

"Taking the time to recognize and celebrate a huge accomplishment is critical to continued success, because it reinforces the passion an athlete must have in order to win a race like the Tour de France," he wrote in an article following the event.

It is very true and, in nearly all my interviews with athletes over the past 25 years, I, too, recognize that one must stop and smell the roses in order to truly appreciate a great achievement.

SECRETS OF SUCCESS: CHRIS WITTY

Chris Witty may be best known as a speed skater, having made light work of her competition in the 2002 Salt Lake City Olympics, where she won the 1000-meter gold medal in long-track speed skating. (This was to add to the collection she brought home 4 years earlier from Nagano as a two-time Olympic medalist: silver in the 1000 meters and bronze in the 1500 meters.)

But Witty isn't just handy with the steel skates; she also rides a mean bicycle, making her one of the most accomplished cross-trainers in US sports. Witty was only the ninth American athlete to compete in Summer and Winter Olympics, having taken her bike to Sydney in 2000. There, she finished fifth in the 500-meter time trial.

"I think the cross-training is good for me, but not for everyone. It keeps me physically tuned and mentally fresh. I'm never doing the same workouts day in and day out," she told me. "I'm always doing something new, and it clears my head. The motor/muscle coordinates are very similar. With speed skating, you support your body and use your ham strings and glutes, and in riding it's the same. Except you don't support your body in riding, you sit. That is the major difference."

Psychologically, it is different, too. "I find myself having to control my body in speed skating, learning certain moves and controlling the turns. Cycling, on the other hand, is more tactical," she declared. "I think if young athletes want to cross-train and compete in both sports, they should do it. It's a treat, and it does keep you mentally refreshed." Here are the issues that Chris Witty says all athletes should be aware of in cross-training.

- Do both sports but keep track of your training; don't overtrain in either place.

- Be careful; there are a lot of crashes in both venues.

- Anticipate a lot of body stress; pay attention.

- Listen to your body; you need to plan your program.

WORKSHEET: MENTAL TRAINING FOR CYCLING

Review these mental training techniques before your next few cycling workouts or races. Customize these tools to meet your individual goals and needs, then note what works for future rides and races.

Use affirmations and self-talk. Practice these during training as well as racing. Tell yourself during a tough race or training ride, "I can do this; I can tough it out." Don't let negative thoughts such as "I'm tiring" or "I don't think I can outsprint this guy" creep in. If you fall off the pack or a rider elbows you or bumps your wheel, tell yourself, "Stay calm; put it behind you." Choose a cue word or phrase such as "You can do it" to use in tough spots during the race.

Breathe right. Practice full breathing regularly (see Chapter 4 for specific practice steps). Before your race, you may want to listen to a specific piece of music to practice relaxed, comfortable breathing. You might pair an image, such as crossing the finish line of the race, with your breathing routine.

Meditate. Meditation during a race or training will help you shut out the outside world and concentrate on your own race. You might choose a mantra such as Kungys': "Looking good, feeling strong, nothing can go wrong!" to repeat before and during the race to help you concentrate and stay relaxed.

Relax. After hard workouts, practice progressive relaxation to ease your muscles. Establish your own relaxation routine with an audiotape. Practice a mini relaxation session using deep breaths or counting backward from 10 to calm yourself if you're getting overly tense during or just before a race.

Practice imagery and visualization. To begin guided imagery, identify how you view images by filling out the questionnaire on page 56. For imagery practice, watch film clips of the Tour de France or other elite races. For inspiration, you might want to rent the classic cycling movie *Breaking Away*. You'll find a guided imagery program on page 240.

Consider your opponents. Lance Armstrong and his coach visualize a varied set of circumstances and other racers at different stages of a competition. It can also help to visualize yourself breaking away from key opponents or winning sprint finishes.

Visualize technique. In your mind, watch yourself cornering, climbing, riding in a pack, breaking away, and sprinting, then slow down your visualization and correct any mistakes you see. Kungys always practices his entire race in his mind before getting to the course. He takes himself through the whole race, feeling the ups and downs of competitive racing, including the enormous amount of fatigue in his quadriceps.

Build a victory image. Kungys's victory images include letting go of his handlebars, raising both hands to the sky, and letting out a sigh of relief. He does this in his mind before each race so that when it's time to win, he'll be ready.

Use visual motor behavior rehearsal (VMBR). Visualize yourself in a race; focus on enhancing your technique and analyzing and mentally correcting errors. While training, practice the corrected behavior. Before races, imagine all the details of the race and how you will meet challenges that might arise. Practice switching back and forth between a relaxed phase and a ready-to-win state of mind (see page 65 for specific steps).

Have a prerace routine. Anticipate, prepare for, and minimize as many distractions as possible. At the race site, check out the surroundings, the crowd, the weather, and the noise. See who your competitors are. Thirty minutes before race time, move into your PTEZ, or perfect timing and energy zone. Practice relaxed breathing. Visualize yourself riding the course, breaking away, dealing with adversity, and finishing strongly. Tell yourself that you will do well in this race. Do any prerace rituals that make you more comfortable. Twigg, for example, uses a ritual of checking equipment on her bike.

CHAPTER 12

Downhill Skiing: See—
Then Ski—Clean Runs

Imagery and visualization training are not optional in the sport of skiing; they're mandatory. Competitive skiers must learn to control all the thoughts and mental pictures cruising around in their minds so that they can have safe, successful runs—not to mention turn in good times. Most ski racers report that they can affect whether they are going to get hurt or not depending on how much mental rehearsal they perform.

After much practice, Olympic skier and three-time World Cup winner Holly Flanders learned how to access her own visual training screen when implementing mental practice strategies. For her, it wasn't just a technique; it was survival.

Flanders took skiing seriously. She trained hard, was diligent about her workouts—both on and off the snow—and practiced a lot of imagery rehearsal. Her coach, Warren Witherell, was influential in helping her focus on imagery skills and many other training strategies in downhill ski racing. In studying her techniques, the core lesson she learned was that the journey of training was just as important as the competition and the results. "What's important is not where you arrive but how you get there," Flanders says.

BUILDING MUSCLE MEMORY

What is muscle memory, and how does it become part of you? Most recreational and competitive skiers watch ski films or videos or televised races, so you've probably seen footage of a ski racer going through a slalom course at high speed. What are the things you look for when you see this blur coming across your screen? First you wonder if that person is going to make it without spilling. Next you question how she ever gets around those turns so fast, perhaps with ice on the course. Third, you focus on the skis, the tips, and the angle at which the skier crosses the downhill slope. You

MENTAL MASTERS

Holly Flanders skied in the 1980 and 1984 Olympics. She was the top American finisher in the downhill in the 1984 Olympics and won World Cup Championships in 1982, 1983, and 1984. Today she is running clinics and doing fund-raisers in her home of Park City, Utah.

Phil Mahre, a three-time Olympian (1976, 1980, and 1984), took a silver medal in the slalom in 1980 and the gold medal in 1984. He cowrote *No Hill Too Steep* with his twin brother, Steve.

Steve Mahre, a three-time Olympian (1976, 1980, and 1984), took a silver medal in the slalom in 1984. Both Steve and Phil Mahre still race in world-class ski competition.

Diann Roffe-Steinrotter, six-time US Champion, was the gold medalist at the World Championship in 1985, a silver medalist in the giant slalom in the 1992 Olympics, and a gold medalist in the 1994 Olympics in the Super G. She is a three-time Olympian.

Stein Eriksen is a legend, especially in his native Norway, where he won gold medals in the 1948 and 1952 Olympics. He also won more medals in the 1950 and 1954 world championships. He presently lives in Deer Valley, Utah, at the Stein Eriksen Lodge.

wonder about how much pressure the ankles and knees can take at that velocity with that G-force. You look for other subtle changes in ski, pole, or body position that signal either good, tight form or loss of control.

Next, you might look at the hips and shoulders, and then you might even look at the goggled face and try to determine an expression of excitement or pain. These are the visual cues that you take in, or digest—all in a matter of seconds—when you see a skilled slalom racer gracing the slopes of a course. You take a visual and kinesthetic inventory to determine all the components of the body in relation to the forces of gravity and nature. This inventory actually gets stored in your brain, like the VCR I mentioned earlier.

These external images go into your internal database and later get shuffled onto your hard drive, along with your internal pictures of how you feel and your level of confidence around downhill skiing. This is the beginning of the mental practice program for skiing. We all do it; it comes naturally, but some of us are just a bit more aware of this internal program than others.

CONFIDENCE BUILDING

Diann Roffe-Steinrotter, who retired from amateur competition after her gold-medal performance in Lillehammer, Norway, at the 1994 Winter Olympics, says she can feel her imagery as well as see it. "I will always watch myself from a video perspective, and that's my kinesthetic, or feeling imagery," she says. "My visual imagery is from within. When I use my visual imagery, I know the sense of confidence and being right there on the course and hitting each gate. Sometimes I combine both my feeling imagery and my visual imagery. That is when I know I am ready to race."

DEALING WITH FATIGUE

With skiing, it's satisfying to know that if you practice, you get better. But it's also important to know that practice is partly physical and partly psychological and emotional. Often when you have a bad run, you might find yourself saying, "I'm tired," "I ate too much lunch," or "I am just burned out for the day." But if you're a racer and you are trying to make the national team, excuses don't cut it. What do racers do when faced with a bad day or just plain fatigue?

Rewind the videotape. Champion Flanders and other great skiers tell us that when the going gets rough, it's time to back up the mental videotape (in your mind's eye) and rerun the program. This time, run the program with a feeling of "I can do it, I have confidence in myself, I know my strengths, and most important, I have been here before." When you back up the mental video, take a few deep breaths and get your body completely relaxed. Significant changes do take place. In other words, you want to combine visual motor rehearsal, deep breathing, and relaxation with positive self-talk and affirmation to get yourself on track, physically and mentally.

Rebuild confidence. First you need to change your attitude. Perhaps you're cold, but you need to remind yourself that you have the strength in your knees, thighs, and ankles to have a great run. Perhaps you are focusing too much energy on one ski. Perhaps you're intimidated by an icy or steep stretch that's prime territory for a skid or fall. That's when it is time to rewind the video, go over the tough place, and visualize in your mind a relaxed, balanced, and comfortable ski through that place. You might even want to mentally rehearse that spot on the chairlift just before tackling it on the slopes. The important thing to remember is to build confidence around your own capabilities and not let images of fear take over.

Take care on those bad days. Recreational skiers as well as Olympic champion racers need to have a sense of their good and bad days, says

---

SECRETS OF SUCCESS:
HOLLY FLANDERS

Train to the Utmost

Holly Flanders, a 1980 and 1984 Olympian, takes her downhill skiing to the max. She pushes the envelope so that she can get the most out of her training. When it's time to race, she knows she has done her homework. The muscle memory is in place; she's ready to go. This has the added benefit of increasing confidence levels.

Roffe-Steinrotter. "If you sense that your timing and emotions are off, pay attention so that you don't do something careless and get injured," she cautions. "There will always be days when your fatigue level is high, and those are days when you do not push the limits. When I'm tired, I fall back on my relaxation and mental rehearsal. I remind myself to relax, take deep breaths, and let my shoulders drop. If I'm about to race, I always go through the same routine: I look ahead, completely focused on the course, let myself hang loose, and think positive thoughts." That's an important caveat. Ski patrollers everywhere will attest to the fact that it tends to be that "one last run of the day" that gets tired skiers into trouble.

Focus, focus. Balance and rhythm can be the deciding factors in an important race, say Flanders and other top skiers. They can also mean the difference between a serious injury or pulling out of something difficult just in time. Many skiers report that preparing themselves for a safe run is just as important as having a fast one. Flanders cautions that most great competitors know that injuries are often brought on when you let yourself become unfocused and out of sync with your training goals.

IMAGERY FOR THE SLOPES

Phil and Steve Mahre, both three-time Olympic skiers, do an enormous amount of imagery work and visualization training. They suggest that all skiers—whether downhill racers or recreational athletes—should constantly train their minds to pick up on visual cues so that they can do effective imagery rehearsal when it is time to ski. Flanders, the Mahre twins, and Roffe-Steinrotter are just a few examples of athletes who have benefited from mental practice strategies in the snow. They recommend that all of us, from neophyte to advanced racer, try mental practice and imagery training, including the tips described below. It can only lead to improved performance and a greater enjoyment of the slopes.

Build a firm foundation. Roffe-Steinrotter and her teammates used to remind each other that every ski run was like depositing money in the bank. "Then, when it comes to race day, you can make withdrawals from that emotional and physical bank," she says. "You are always building the blocks as part of the psychological training foundation."

See yourself on the snow. Flanders is now a ski instructor in Park City, Utah, and she reminds others learning to ski that training has two components. "The first is what you do on the slopes; the second (and equally important) is what you do off the slopes. Sometimes when you do dry-land training or cross-training away from the snow, such as cycling and balance-board work, the most important ingredient is to see yourself on the snow, moving your hips and shifting your weight and in the perfect rhythm of downhill skiing."

Inspect the course. Roffe-Steinrotter is scientific about her skiing, especially when it comes to international competition. She always takes plenty of time to inspect the course, first riding up the chair to take a look and then sliding down the course to feel it firsthand. "I look at all aspects of the terrain—the flats, where it rolls, the rough spots, and where the snow might be choppy," she says. "To be a great skier, you have to memorize each set of gates in every part of the hill. I always slid down with a coach or another athlete, and then I went off from everyone, hid out, and started to imagine my ski run." Phil Mahre suggests that you inspect all aspects of a slope or race course, including the snow conditions. This includes a visual inspection in person, followed by a mental run-through in your mind 15 to 20 times before you even put your skis on. As you ride the chairlift or after you suit up in the lodge, study the trail map, mentally rehearsing the run you plan to take after you reach the summit.

Pay special attention to gates. In a slalom race, Phil Mahre recommends that you go from the bottom to the top of the mountain, stopping at specific gates to get a good mental picture of the slope and the individual turns. Mahre was known to hike up five gates and then run through those five gates in his mind. He then hiked another eight, ran through those gates mentally and then hiked seven more, and so on. He always memorized where it got steeper, where it was flatter, where the combinations were, and what the snow conditions were. Mahre looked at whether the gates were on a roll or back from that roll so that he could anticipate where he might lose some pressure with the ski. "With skiing, it's a visual recall phenomenon," Mahre points out. "And that recall of images triggers the feeling part so that you can put weight and pressure on your skis at the gate at just the right moment. Amateur competitors can do the same thing with the NASTAR [National Standard Race] courses set up at major ski areas."

Use self-talk. The trick to good skiing for both racers and recreational athletes is to not talk yourself into a fall, says Phil Mahre. "Often you see a spot that might look bad from the chairlift, and you start visualizing catastrophic events. Or, while skiing, you see an icy patch or deep rut a few turns ahead and think, 'Uh-oh, I'm going to fall.'" Then you do. Mahre reminds us that, right from the start, you can't have any negative thoughts. "Negative thoughts often lead to apprehension, which then contributes to muscle tension. If that happens, you are headed for danger and possible injury. To counter that tension, you have to remind yourself to relax. You have to do self-talk and tell yourself to be relaxed on the ice and to maintain a positive and confident attitude," says Mahre. "As soon as you start backing off any turn, any slope, you are going to tighten your body, lose form, and take a spill."

Erase negative images. Steve Mahre used imagery as if it were part of a daily ritual. His most vivid images of successful ski racing took him to a place in Europe, to a very tough downhill course he had to conquer. "I was in the German Alps. I was at the starting gate, and there was one spot on the ski course that I was unfamiliar with," he says. "I didn't feel very confident about it, and I knew that it wasn't feeling right. I went down the course and fell right in the place I had been thinking about. It's as if I had locked into a negative image on that one turn. I just couldn't seem to undo that program in my mind. And once I fell, I was fine. It was now out of my system, off the mental picture screen. Now I was ready to race again; I just had to remove and erase that bad visual image."

Be ready for distractions. For Roffe-Steinrotter, getting focused and staying in the present was an art form. Sometimes, after a major spill, getting up and refocusing toward a positive outcome can be the most challenging part of the whole event. "The day before the Olympic Super G in 1994, I scared myself with a big spill against the fence," she says. "It was a practice run, and I got hurt, so I had to psych myself up and reorient myself to a positive frame of mind. I had a sense of uncertainty about the start of the Olympics. I was already set in my visualization for a great competition, but now I had to factor in this other variable. You have to expect these little distractions and know how to deal with them. After this little episode, my husband, who was also my part-time coach, was fond of saying that when I got ready to race, there was 'more sparkle in my eye and more fire under my butt.' He knew I was ready."

Prepare to avoid injury. Many skiers such as Flanders know about the relationship of imbalance or unfocused training to injury. "Unless you are really strong psychologically and really committed to staying healthy, you

SECRETS OF SUCCESS:
PHIL MAHRE

Seek Out the Edge

As a champion Olympic racer, Phil Mahre notes that aggressiveness is really important, or you tend to lose your focus. "You have to take those chances, which is all about being on the edge, if not over the edge," he says. "You find that line for yourself, and then that's where you push yourself to. You're right on the threshold, and as time goes by, that threshold gets higher and higher and higher with better training."

can get injured so easily in ski racing, because in an injury-causing situation, you don't have much time to think and react," she says. "It has to be instinctive—already a part of your muscle memory developed through training. You have to work on it psychologically and emotionally. In ski racing, it's very important to visualize everything. We use visualization every moment of our training, and if you incorporate the wrong mental pictures, you can get into some very serious trouble."

Analyze errors and good runs alike. Roffe-Steinrotter and her Olympic cohorts used a lot of videotape to observe their training runs, styles, and techniques. Their video training sessions were broken down into slow-motion and freeze-frame segments as well as real time. Roffe-Steinrotter enjoyed watching the full-speed action of her downhill so that she could plug it into her kinesthetic hard drive. "I always spent lots of time by myself watching videos of my skiing," she says. "When you have a good day on the slopes, you don't always know how or why it was so good. Not until you see the video do you know the magic of that day."

WHEN THINGS GO WRONG

Roffe-Steinrotter says that the first thing that comes to mind when she considers mental rehearsal is mental toughness. "If you haven't struggled or had a rough time with your skiing, then you won't understand how to structure your training," she says. "You can tell a 17-year-old that she needs to practice mental skills, but if she has not struggled with her sport, she simply won't believe you."

Roffe-Steinrotter believes that many elite-level athletes take their sports for granted, especially ski racing, until D day. That's the day you hit the Wall, that feeling of fatigue and sense of doom, and blow out a knee or have a serious accident—a turning point in most careers. That is the day when you face your vulnerability as a mortal athlete. That day usually begins the process of surgery and a long road back through rehabilitation and recovery. "That is when you learn what you are made of and the next level of commitment you must make to be the best," says Roffe-Steinrotter.

In the late 1980s, Roffe-Steinrotter went from second in the world rankings to 60th in a matter of months. She had 18 knee injuries, and her fitness level changed dramatically. Her work ethic was mediocre, and her attitude about training was poor. She didn't understand what she needed to do to get strong. She was facing a crisis (and a turning point) in her ski career. Right before the 1988 Olympics, she made a conscious decision to change her lifestyle and move back home to spend more time with her family. She decided to start a new training program that included more mental and physical discipline. "I had to approach things in a new way, with new expectations for my performance level. I had to start feeling good about myself and my work ethic. Initially, my success was due to raw talent and being feisty, but as you get older, the pressure is greater and that style doesn't always cut it. You need a training base and discipline with a schedule."

Injuries have been a big part of Roffe-Steinrotter's life. She tore an anterior cruciate ligament in her knee in 1990 and was treated by renowned surgeon, Richard Steadman, MD, of Vail, Colorado. Seven months after surgery, she started skiing again. She made a dramatic change in her life and her attitude toward training. She was committed to trying harder, complaining less, and having a stronger work ethic. She had to put fear on the back burner and not worry about getting reinjured. Her rehab was a combination of physical and emotional training, including a lot of time in the pool working with a flotation belt.

"I tried to get in the pool every day and do the stairclimber and the stationary bike," says Roffe-Steinrotter. "The big thing was stretching and

SECRETS OF SUCCESS:
STEIN ERIKSEN

Stein Eriksen is a legend in the ski world, both in the United States and around the world, especially in his native Norway, where he won gold medals in the 1948 and 1952 Olympics. He won more medals in the 1950 and 1954 world championships. In fact, in 2004, Stein was honored in Norway at the 50-year reunion of the world team. At 75, he still is a graceful, lively, and incredibly talented skier.

But he may never have achieved his goals if his parents hadn't approached his skills with the right mix of encouragement and support.

"My father was a great skier; he taught me all about it, but he didn't push. He let me have the space to grow with competition, without forcing me to compete," Eriksen says. "He and my mother embraced my sport and empowered me to become a great champion, but they did not push; they stayed on the sidelines. Too many kids get pushed and overloaded by parents living vicariously, and they burn out. My son is 23, and he skis very well, plays tennis and golf extremely well, but he does not want to compete. So I say to him enjoy your sport, enjoy the outdoors, and improve every day, but don't force yourself to be a competitor."

Tips from Stein Eriksen:

- Children who ski need to be trained in gymnastics. Conditioning and flexibility is essential for quality skiing.

- Inspiration comes from mothers and fathers; they can help.

- Ability and agility are equally important. Slalom skiing involves maneuvers—flexibility, concentration.

- Cross-train with tennis. It builds in concentration as it teaches focus.

mentally rehearsing a healthy ski run. Relaxation and reading between workouts were very important. You have to learn how to relax and let down emotionally to help you deal with the stress of racing. You need to call on that relaxation period at all times."

WORKSHEET: MENTAL TRAINING
FOR DOWNHILL SKIING

Review these mental training techniques before your next race or training run. You'll want to customize this program to meet your own goals and needs and take note of what images or techniques work best for you.

Use affirmations and self-talk. Practice these during training as well as racing. Tell yourself during a tough race or workout, "I can do this" or "Stay relaxed; stay confident." Don't allow negative thoughts, such as worrying about a tough spot on the course or thinking about falling. If you have a bad start, a poor turn, or a fall, put it behind you and look ahead. Use a cue word or phrase such as "You can do it" during tough spots in the competition.

Breathe right. Practice full breathing regularly (see Chapter 4 for specific practice steps). If you race, you may want to listen to a specific piece of music to practice relaxed, comfortable breathing. You might pair an image, such as crossing the finish line, with your breathing routine. Even if you're not racing, remember to breathe. Time your breaths with the rhythm of your pole plants. Otherwise, you may find yourself holding your breath, which creates muscle tension and deprives your muscles of needed oxygen.

Meditate. Meditation during a race or training will help you shut out the outside world and concentrate on your own race. You may choose to repeat to yourself, "Stay relaxed; keep positive and confident," as Phil Mahre likes to remind himself. Repeat your mantra before and during the race to help yourself concentrate and stay relaxed. If you're skiing recreationally, use the ride up the lift or gondola to focus on one word or simple image, blocking out distractions.

Relax. After hard workouts, practice progressive relaxation to relax your muscles. Establish your own relaxation routine with an audiotape. Practice relaxing during workouts so that you can call up the relaxation response during races, if needed. The ride up the chairlift is the perfect opportunity to use progressive relaxation to dissipate tension that accumulates in your neck, arms, chest, back, legs, and especially your feet.

Practice imagery and visualization. To begin guided imagery, identify how you view images by filling out the questionnaire on page 56. For imagery practice, watch film clips of races or instructional videos. Visualize the good days as well as the bad ones. Remember that conditions play a big part in how you react to a tough situation, so visualize a blizzard and hard-driving race conditions, then switch gears to see a blue sky with fresh powder. Know yourself in both sets of conditions. You'll find a guided imagery program on page 240.

Consider your opponents. You'll have to experiment to see if this is helpful to you. Olympic medalist Picabo Street is tough and imagines no competition, even though she can see other opponents. She rarely sees an opponent because she only visualizes herself, several seconds out front on the giant slalom.

Visualize technique. Technique is crucial for skiing. Pole position, staying forward on your skis, knee and ankle angulation, carving, and full-line positioning all require constant focus for a clear run, whether your goal is to ski fast or just cruise.

Build a victory image. Tommy Moe, an Olympic gold medalist, was so good at winning that there was some question as to whether he knew how to lose a downhill race. "I always picture myself on the victory podium when I practice my races," he told a reporter, "so that I can't imagine ending up anyplace else."

Use visual motor behavior rehearsal (VMBR). Visualize yourself in a race; focus on enhancing your technique and analyzing and mentally correcting errors. In your mind, watch yourself during a race or run and slow down your visualization and correct any mistakes you see. If your turns have been a little sloppy—not quite clean or complete—visualize the ski flexing and hugging the snow as it curves. Visualize the shadow you make as you cruise downhill, around turns, and over moguls in perfect ski form. While training, practice the corrected behavior. Before races, image all the details of the race and how you will meet challenges that might arise. Practice switching back and forth between a relaxed phase and a ready-to-win state of mind (see page 65 for specific steps).

Have a prerace routine. Anticipate, prepare for, and minimize as many distractions as possible. At the race site, check out the surroundings, the crowd, the weather, and the noise. Look around to see who your competitors are. Thirty minutes before race time, move into your PTEZ, or perfect timing and energy zone. Practice relaxed breathing; visualize yourself skiing the course, making each turn, dealing with adversity, and finishing strongly. Tell yourself that you will do well in this race. Do any prerace rituals that make you more comfortable.

If you're skiing recreationally, anticipate obstacles and distractions that you'll be apt to encounter—slower skiers, patches of thin cover, spray from snow guns, trail debris. Before your run, adjust your boot buckles, secure your hat and goggles, and warm up your hands; but once you start your run, put those things out of your mind and focus on the course. I've been a strong recreational skier for 40 years and have always relied on straightedge downhill skis. When my friend and coach Doug Harcleroad encouraged me to try his parabolics, I was hesitant. But it turned out they make carving and turning more fun and a bit easier. Of course, they are not for everyone — you have to find the equipment that works well for you.

CHAPTER 13

Golf: Set the Stage
for Excellence

During the 1992 Olympic Games in Barcelona, rumor had it that the Dream Team—composed largely of US basketball superstars—wasn't visiting Spain just to play basketball. Michael Jordan, for one, played golf incessantly during his stay. Jordan got teased about his early morning forays, but the fact remains that the golf course is the one place he could go to really relax and get away from the pressures of Olympic competition.

Golf indeed can be an emotionally forgiving sport. Many athletes, both professional and recreational, note that golf is the one sport that allows them to be physically relaxed and yet mentally focused when they escape their other obligations in the world. In 1924, C. W. Bailey wrote a book titled *The Brain and Golf: Some Hints for Golfers from Modern Mental Science*, which begins by telling the reader that the "mind is the master of muscle." There is a suggestion that modern science "may actually help players improve their game of golf." Bailey goes on to note in his introduction: "Swinging a club both indoors and outside on a regular basis will enhance balance, rhythm, and accuracy of movement, and lead to a more stable golf game. The lesson of this mental science of golf is that the most consistent game is played by the aid of the subconscious mind, so the function of golf exercise is to make certain necessary movements as automatic as possible."

HOW A LEGEND DOES IT

Almost 70 years later, in an article in *Golf* magazine, Jack Nicklaus shared almost identical insights about his strongest weapon—the power of his mind to influence a strong golf game. Nicklaus claims that although he was one of the longest straight drivers and an excellent pressure putter, his strongest asset was his mind. "Your mind should always be your strongest weapon in your game," he said in the article. "However, if you suspect that your head is your enemy, there are some techniques that will help you shift to a positive attitude."

Nicklaus's first rule is to assess how you see yourself as a golfer. What is the image that you have? Do you see yourself as just swinging and ball striking? For Nicklaus, the key has been to mentally prepare before each swing instead of focusing on just a golf score. Nicklaus always goes with a swing that he has rehearsed and used for years; he does not experiment on the course. He uses a warmup swing and then records the thought that goes with that warmup so that he can take that into his actual golf stroke.

Nicklaus has said that "even at the highest levels of golf, perfect shots are mostly accidental and extremely rare." Is this really one of the greatest

MENTAL MASTERS

Jeff Quinney went to Arizona State University and played Division I golf all 4 years, from 1997 to 2001, capping off his collegiate career with being the US amateur champion in 2000.

Peter Jacobsen is one of the most successful PGA players in America today. He has been on the pro tour for nearly 3 decades and has won just about every major tournament.

Chuck Hogan, a professional golfer, has been a coach since 1989. He has coached Peter Jacobsen, Johnny Miller, Ray Floyd, Mike Reid, Duffy Waldorf, and Mark Wiebe.

Steve Nosler has been the head golf coach at the University of Oregon in Eugene for more than 11 years and has been involved with competitive golf since the 1960s.

golf experts speaking? What he means by this comment is that we all have talent, some a bit more than others. On any given day we all might hit one perfect shot, but the great golfer distinguishes himself from the average ones by reducing the severity of misses. Learning to manage your missed shots is really the greatest asset to the mental game of golf.

Like Nicklaus, Arnold Palmer, and other golf greats, many of us possess terrific potential. Most of us have a unique blend of innate drive matched with ability, but we also have a tendency to interfere with our strengths. We often interfere with our own abilities to perform and learn the game of golf. Because we all have moments of greatness, it is frustrating and often exasperating when we realize that we will not always have our best stroke on the course.

FOCUS, THEN RELAX

Many golfers suggest that intense focus and unwavering concentration are the only ways to approach a serious golf game. Others might argue that if you only had that singular, one-dimensional focus, you would become extremely tired and mentally fatigued at the end of 18 holes. Palmer, Nicklaus, and others often suggest moving from one intensely focused arena to a "valley of relaxation" as needed; that is, experiencing your golf game as a two-tiered state of being—first, learning how to focus intensely, and second, learning how and when to let down and move into a complete state of relaxation. By moving between both phases—the focus followed by complete relaxation—you allow yourself to complete a full cycle of intensity and then a break from the intensity, or active rest.

Nicklaus has written extensively about this notion of intense focus followed by active rest. In *Golf* magazine, he discussed his complete concentration beginning when he arrives at the tee. The focus becomes more intense as he completes his process of analysis and evaluation for his shot. He gets to his next level, "the ultimate focal point," when he sets up to the ball and executes his swing. At this point, Nicklaus and other great golfers have a clear visual image of the perfect swing, followed by the perfect shot, followed by the perfect outcome. These are all strong visual images that emerge from years of practice both on the course and in the mind's eye before getting to the greens.

Immediately following this intense focal period, most golfers let themselves off the hook for a moment. They also let their minds wander to the crowd, listen to noises, and engage in brief conversation or even think about something unrelated to golf. This is the active rest period. This is when you give yourself permission for a bit of R & R so that you can have quiet time before you gear up mentally for the next round of intense focus and concentration.

Jeff Quinney, a former US amateur champion and relatively new pro, testifies that alternating between focus and relaxation is still a popular mental practice among golfers today, including himself.

"When you walk from the tee to the ball, it's okay to wander emotionally, but you need to refocus when it's time to hit. I talk to my caddy for a

SECRETS OF SUCCESS: JEFF QUINNEY

Jeff Quinney offers these tips.

- Balance your work and athleticism, your social life and golf life.

- Set goals for your game.

- When you travel a lot or you have a lot of free time, you have to build structure and manage your time well and practice with quality.

- Don't obsess with your game: Try to avoid 24/7 golf. Go to movies, go to the mall, release the pressure of the game, go out with people who are not golfers, and don't talk the game all day long.

- Golf is such a mental game that it takes up lots of time. You need a good instructor and years of practice, and you need to start early.

- If you get injured, get a good physical therapist. Do lots of stretching and ease back into the game.

- While in rehab, watch lots of video, break down your game and your strokes, and use the video as another pair of eyes to improve your visual game. "Video really helps me see everything more clearly; it helps me with correcting my shot," Quinney says.

healthy distraction, but I don't wander too far from my game," he explained to me. "My goal is hit, let go emotionally, and then refocus for the next shot. Don't get caught in reliving the stroke or the putt. Let go of it!"

Here's how professionals gear up for this focus period.

Do your advance work. Peter Jacobsen, winner of the 2003 Greater Hartford Open, suggests playing the course in your mind before you begin. "I always run through it visually; I visualize the shots and what clubs I will use," he says. "Everything is done in advance so I know exactly what and where I'm going before I get to the links. If the greens are thick, I need to visualize that and feel that in order to recover from a particular shot."

Control distractions. Professional golfer and coach Chuck Hogan explains that problems in golf occur when you make errors in target selection and club selection and when major distractions away from the course pull you away from your game. "Golfers are usually saturated with excess baggage," he says. Mental training can help you learn to let go of those distractions and clear your mind before competitions.

Treat it like a game. Many golfers will testify to the fact that you cannot force the game. You cannot make a shot happen. You must release the self-imposed pressure by thinking of golf as just a game—and a fun one at that. Nicklaus tells a story of reading the novels of renowned author W. Somerset Maugham and coming away with a different attitude about life and perhaps his approach to golf. Maugham suggested that one enjoy life with an "amused tolerance," and Nicklaus says he has tried to implement that philosophy in his golf game. If you allow yourself that amused tolerance that Nicklaus derived from Maugham, you might play better and enjoy the game more.

Ride out the cycles. Golf is that roller coaster of emotions. On the one hand, when we play well, there is a sense of wonderment and even some fantasies about how great we might someday become. On the other hand, we can have three perfect rounds followed by a week of terrible golf. It is this continual cycle of emotional highs and lows that seduces us into wanting to play, master, and even control the game. There lies the problem. Control is a big issue. If you try to control your game, chances are that you will have dismal outcomes.

Focus ahead of time. "There is a great deal of slippage between intention and behavior in this subtle game of golf," says Hogan. "And what I mean is, you cannot have ambiguities in this game. You have to have clear intention and clear focus before you hit the greens."

SECRETS OF SUCCESS:
PETER JACOBSEN

Peter Jacobsen loves to inject fun into his game to take the edge off. Here are his suggestions.

- Design a positive distraction when you play and compete. "I like to engage with other athletes," Jacobsen says.

- Write down your love and passions: cars, movies, literature, football, etc. Talk about and think about those on the course.

- Take breaks from golf occasionally. Do other sports—anything that's fun.

- Limit your negative comments. It takes awhile to get good at golf. Remind yourself of that when things get tough.

HARNESSING YOUR EMOTIONS

W. Timothy Gallwey, best-selling author of *The Inner Game of Golf*, has some interesting insights for people just beginning golf. When Gallwey first began to play, he played in a celebrity golf tournament in Los Angeles and was paired with a famous brain surgeon. The surgeon, identified only as Dr. F., was having a rough day on the course and on several occasions slammed his driver to the ground, proclaiming that golf was the most frustrating game ever invented. After an hour of complete exasperation and more tantrums, Gallwey recounted that he asked the doctor why he played if it frustrated him so much. The noted surgeon commented, "It is the only game I play that I can't beat!"

Gallwey learned from this experience and his own frustration on the course that golf is indeed a very seductive sport. It is a sport that brings out the best in men and women, and the worst. It is a sport that in a hot flash of anger we promise to quit, followed a few moments later by a complete ego gratification with the perfect putt. After all, golf has a bit of luck attached to it; you can play for years and never achieve that inner sanctum of success and deep fulfillment.

Here are some tips to help you find your path to your best and most rewarding golf game.

Use mental practice to tune up. "We all start with a similar physical and talent base, a certain minimum technique and a standard of performance," says Steve Nosler, head golf coach at the University of Oregon in Eugene. "The mental practice, the visualization, and the self-image side of the golf game come later as a fine-tuning to the physiological component. It doesn't change the game so much as build on confidence and ego strengths."

Take a look at yourself. The best way to analyze your swing and grip is to view yourself on videotape, says Nosler. Get a friend with a video camera to film you on the links and watch the video carefully, pinpointing mistakes.

Let mistakes go. Experts tell us that the game of golf is not so much about control as it is about self-control. That is, golf is about learning to ride out the emotions—the roller coaster of ups and downs on any given day on the course. If we can learn to let go of the bad shots and embrace the beautiful, picture-perfect ones, these emotional waves will balance out in the overall scheme of the game. If we can learn to ride out the storm as well as play consistently during the calm, we will indeed have a better handle on our inner self-control and enhance the quality of play. If his golfers hit the trees, Nosler tells them not to worry about it and to move ahead. "I try to empower my athletes to find the right mental attitude while I provide the technical side," he says. "I don't try to force anything on my athletes; the game is a passive game of active concentration."

Clear your mind. "Golf is very much like life," says Nosler. "It is a very sensitive game; each day is precious, and you have to set the stage for excellence each day. If you have distractions in your mind, your game will suffer." If Nosler finds that he isn't getting any response from a golfer he is coaching, he'll often find that the golfer is being distracted by other problems. "Then we have to address those issues that are affecting the flow and balance of the golf game," he explains.

Picture the shot. Most golfers—weekend duffers and touring pros alike—will attest to the fact that you can't really hit a good shot without having a clear mental picture of it before you swing. In golf, this is a must. For some, the golf ball and swing is like a beautiful ballet of image and form with the backdrop of grass and trees to fill in the collage of this perfect mental image. For many, the image of the ball shooting into space followed by the perfect landing on the course is part of the ideal visualization.

Give it your all. Hogan says that there's no separate mental side to golf. "What you see in a golfer is all mental," he says. "You don't compartmentalize it into 65 percent physical, 35 percent mental. That is not what this sport is about. If you believe in the mental versus the physical, then you're in trouble. It means that you have split yourself into two beings. And if you split yourself, you are not a whole person; you're two halves struggling for continuity and completeness in this very sensitive game known as golf."

Don't overanalyze. Hogan says that we intellectualize the game of golf to death and don't understand that it is quite simple. "The game is about the human experience on the course; you don't have to psychoanalyze every aspect of it," he says. "I think that it is misleading to try and break out all the mental pieces of the game."

Aim for the zone. For Hogan, an athlete is really playing great golf when he is in the zone—the peak performance zone, or what I call the perfect timing and energy zone. This is a place golfers report as being very easy and where they play with a suspension of the conscious mind. "Golfers in the zone are very passive in their conscious minds, and you can never get

SECRETS OF SUCCESS: STEVE NOSLER

Fine-Tuning Your Game

Golf coach Steve Nosler offers these tips.

- Sixty percent of practice time should be in chipping and putting.

- Hitting the driver is fun, but it will not enhance your game.

- To finish strongly, you must start well.

- Practice the sand bunkers, the pitch shot, and other short work.

- When your game needs fine-tuning, bring in outside experts.

them to quantify that state of being. They just know that there is a sense of serenity and safety in their game."

WORKSHEET: MENTAL TRAINING FOR GOLF

Review these mental training techniques before your next golf game or practice session. You'll want to customize these tools to meet your own goals and needs and take note of what images or techniques work best for you.

Use affirmations and self-talk. Do these during practice as well as in games. Tell yourself during a tough game, "I can do this." Don't allow negative thoughts such as "Those other golfers are better than I am" or "I don't think I can make this shot." If you have a bad start or hit a ball into the rough, stay calm and concentrate on moving on. Choose a cue word or phrase such as "You can do it" to use in tough spots during the competition.

Breathe right. Practice full breathing regularly (see Chapter 4 for specific practice steps). Before your game, you may want to listen to a specific piece of music to practice relaxed, comfortable breathing. You might pair an image, such as sinking the ball cleanly into the hole, with your breathing routine.

Meditate. Meditation during a game or practice will help you shut out the outside world and concentrate on your own efforts. You might choose a mantra such as "Stay calm, stay cool" to repeat before and during the game to help you concentrate and stay relaxed.

Relax. After hard workouts, practice progressive relaxation to relax your muscles. Establish your own relaxation routine with an audiotape. Practice a mini relaxation session, perhaps using deep breaths or counting backward from 10 to calm yourself or relax overly tense muscles, say, in your neck. Practice relaxing during workouts so that you can call up the relaxation response during competition, if needed.

Practice imagery and visualization. To begin guided imagery, identify how you view images by filling out the questionnaire on page 56. For imagery practice, watch film clips of professional golfers during competitions that you tape on your VCR, or watch instructional golfing videos that you can find at sporting goods stores. Visualize yourself competing and doing well. In your mind, watch yourself playing golf and slow down your visualization and correct any mistakes you see. You'll find a guided imagery program on page 240.

Consider your opponents. Golf is so individual that imaging an opponent could be counterproductive for you. Nicklaus notes that you can only play against yourself and the course, so preparing mentally might include visualizing the course as your major opponent.

Visualize technique. Watch yourself playing, studying each aspect of your game. Watch how you grip the club, how you position your feet and hands, and how you pivot as you swing.

Build a victory image. The game of golf is won and lost with scant millimeters, so while you practice your stroke, practice how it feels to stand in front of a crowd, smiling broadly as you just birdied your 18th hole. Check out that wonderful feeling.

Use visual motor behavior rehearsal (VMBR). Visualize yourself in a tournament; focus on enhancing your technique and analyzing and mentally correcting errors. While training, practice the corrected behavior. Before competitions or even friendly games, imagine all the details of the event and how you will meet challenges that might arise. Practice switching back and forth between a relaxed phase and a ready-to-win state of mind (see page 65 for specific steps).

Have a precompetition routine. Anticipate, prepare for, and minimize as many distractions as possible. At the golf course, check out the surroundings, the crowd, the weather, and the noise. Thirty minutes before tee time, move into your PTEZ, or perfect timing and energy zone. Practice relaxed breathing; visualize yourself dealing with adversity and finishing strongly. Tell yourself that you will do well in this competition. Do any pre-event rituals that make you more comfortable. Nosler tells his golfers to use their natural ability, relax their forearms, and have fun on the course. According to the great golfers, such as Nicklaus and Palmer, you have to leave all your baggage behind when you hit the links. When you get prepared to play your best golf, let go of any mental baggage, any distractions, and any thoughts that might take your mind from complete focus on the game.

CHAPTER 14

Marathoning: Run Your Best Race Ever

At the height of the running boom in the early 1980s, nearly 25 million people of all ages, shapes, and sizes were running marathons. Olympic gymnast Kathy Johnson (now Johnson-Clarke) trained and ran a marathon to stay in shape and to enjoy the camaraderie that exists among runners. Lynn Swann, the great Pittsburgh Steeler receiver, ran the New York City Marathon in 1993 just to experience the Big Apple. World-class steeplechaser Kelly Jensen, after being out of competitive running for 7 years, set a goal of joining the other 25,000 runners at the 1991 New York City Marathon—and not only did so but also finished in a respectable 2 hours and 38 minutes. Years ago, I ran my first marathon in the heat and oppressive humidity of Honolulu. Along with 30,000 other people, I got up at 4:00 a.m. and jogged to the start in pitch black. It was a bonding experience for all of us, especially since I knew that I was not going to finish in grand style. It was a partylike atmosphere, with folks along the route spraying us with hoses and offering us cold drinks. My second marathon, the Nike Oregon one, was a different story. There I trained and set very specific goals and finished strong (albeit, with cramps).

Suffice it to say, running marathons is an amazing test of an athlete's will and perseverance, but competing in a marathon and even finishing one is a very realistic goal, provided you prepare yourself for the physical and mental rigors. Amby Burfoot, executive editor of *Runner's World* magazine, well-published author, and winner of the 1968 Boston Marathon, says: "It takes enormous discipline, focus, and preparation—both physical and mental—to compete in a marathon." Burfoot, who has been covering marathons across the globe as well as running them, notes, "At any age and at any stage of competition, you must have a game plan."

A WINNER WITH A DREAM

Mark Plaatjes had a dream—a persistent, clearly articulated visual dream—to compete against (and, ultimately, outrace) the best runners in the world. But as a South African, he was barred from competing internationally. It wasn't until 1992, when he became a US citizen, that he had the chance to see his dream to reality.

But just having dreams wouldn't make them come true. Plaatjes had a systematic formula for winning that race. He knew his goals, knew the course, and visualized every aspect of the race.

Plaatjes is the ultimate marathon athlete and the ultimate mentally prepared athlete: He is the complete package. He knew that to be competitive at the 1993 Track and Field World Championship in Stuttgart, Germany, he had to prepare physically and psychologically. He had to run hard and train hard under all kinds of conditions. He also knew that to be a winner, he had to cover all his bases, both physiologically and emotionally.

But as a licensed physical therapist, Plaatjes is cautious about his training techniques. He knows about stress and strain, pulls and tears, and how to prevent all the potential nightmares that befall most great marathoners. He knows how hard to push on his training runs in the hills of Boulder. He also knows when to rest and when to cross-train in a pool, on a bike, or on a stairclimber.

To maximize his training without risking injury, Plaatjes turns to mental practice. "I know that there are major psychological components that one must pay attention to when racing internationally," he told me from his home in Boulder. "For one, you have to have a confidence base. You build confidence not only by getting your miles in but also by training according to your projected hours on the course. If you expect to run a 3-hour marathon, for example, you had better get out there and experience the psychology and physiology of a 3-hour run."

MENTAL MASTERS

Christine Clark, MD, won the 2000 US Olympic Trials and was awarded the sole women's marathon spot to compete in Sydney at the Olympic Games. Her time at the trials was a blistering 2 hours, 33 minutes, 31 seconds.

Amby Burfoot won the Boston Marathon in 1968 and has been executive editor of *Runner's World* for the past 20 years.

Benji Durden was a member of the US Olympic Marathon Team in 1980. He won the 1981 Nike Marathon and beat Bill Rodgers to win the 1982 Houston Marathon. His personal record (PR) is a 2:09:58 in Boston in 1983. He lives in Boulder, Colorado, where he coaches other marathoners.

Hal Higdon was the first American finisher at the Boston Marathon in 1964. In 1981 he won the World Veterans' Championship with a 2:29 at the age of 49. He writes for *Runner's World* magazine and has written several books on running, including *Run Fast, Marathon,* and *Boston,* a history of the Boston Athletic Association Marathon.

Kim Jones placed second in the Boston Marathon in 1991 and 1993, second in the New York City Marathon in 1989 and 1990, fifth at the 1988 Olympic Trials, and eighth at the 1993 World Championship in Stuttgart, Germany. Her PR is a 2:26:40 in Boston in 1991.

Don Kardong finished fourth at the 1976 Olympics in Montreal with a PR of 2:11:16. He won the Honolulu Marathon in 1978.

Kenny Moore was a member of the 1968 and 1972 Olympic Marathon Teams and has won numerous running awards. He is a senior writer for *Sports Illustrated.*

Mark Plaatjes ran a 2:13:57 to win the 1993 World Marathon Championship 3 weeks after he became an American citizen. His best time of 2:08:58 was in 1985. Plaatjes is now a physical therapist who practices in Boulder, Colorado. He was the first American man to win a major marathon since Greg Meyer won at Boston in 1983.

Before running in Germany, the most important race of his life, Plaatjes discussed the course with other athletes, studying the turns, the hills, and the contours. A group of Japanese marathoners who came to Colorado to train before the World Championship shared with him a book filled with notes about various components of the Stuttgart Marathon course. "They had charted every environmental aspect over the past several years," said Plaatjes.

He also prepared for the pack itself. "My training partner helped me prepare for the pack of runners—the feeling of being trapped," he explained. "In your daily training you can't prepare physically for something like a crowd, but you certainly can get ready mentally to cope with it!"

To help prepare for race conditions, Plaatjes ran four races in humid and hot conditions. "I know that heat is a problem for me, so I visualized heat. I even sat in saunas after every training run so that I could simulate a very hot condition. I knew that there would be hills and turns, so I went to courses with hills and turns. I also constantly visualized these contours in my brain so that I was thoroughly prepared. I went out and ran the Peachtree course in Atlanta. It's hot and hilly, so it was a good simulation."

When Plaatjes toured the Stuttgart course before the race, it was like revisiting somewhere he had already been, thanks to his preparation.

After winning his gold medal as an American citizen, Plaatjes had actualized a 15-year-old dream. "I dreamed of being an American, I dreamed of racing internationally, and I dreamed constantly of winning that gold medal," he said.

THE MARATHON IN YOUR MIND

Olympic marathoner Don Kardong tells a wonderful story, one that illustrates a great lesson. During a training run in high school, his coach told him that there was a place on the cross-country course that all competitors would aim for. It was a patch of dirt that looked like a shortcut to the finish but in fact only saved 2 feet. Kardong's coach told him to stay on the pavement and not stray to the dirt path, even though it looked like a faster route.

"He was so sure of himself. He drilled that spot into my mind, and I visualized that mark for weeks," says Kardong. "My coach told me, 'When the others take the shortcut, you start your kick to the finish.' It was the benchmark—the environmental cue to make a move." The combination of the confidence that his coach instilled in him and the visual rehearsals really tapped into his innermost mind-body functions. "I won my first cross-country race that day, and it was the most important training experience of my life. Those images of that place on the course and my coach's voice will be part of me forever."

Here are some insights from Kardong and other top marathoners and coaches about working mental training into your marathoning regimen.

Get your head ready. Kardong believes that there is one crucial element for any athlete, whether recreational or elite, who switches from training for shorter races, such as the 10-K, to training for the marathon. The marathon distance, he says, is strictly a mental game. "The physiological training is not that different at 26 miles. There's some more weekly mileage, but the work needs to be done in your head," he says. "The mental practice before you train for that distance will greatly enhance how your body copes with the stress."

Build your plan well in advance. Longtime marathoner Hal Higdon, who writes for *Runner's World* magazine and has written several books on running, including *Run Fast*, *Marathon*, and *Boston*, attributes his longevity in marathoning to following a specific training routine and having a healthy respect for the distance. In 1992, he perhaps got a bit carried away, running six marathons on six consecutive weekends at the age of 60. Higdon says that the beauty of the marathon is not the running of the event but the preparation and goal setting that goes into the race. "I feel that the motivation and discipline that both recreational and elite athletes set forth in achieving their goals for a marathon is the most important part of the event," he says. "The marathon is about structure: structure in training, diet, attitude, and physical and mental preparation. One usually sets out a plan 6 to 9 months in advance when he or she prepares to go the 26.2 miles. For disciplined folks, the marathon is a way to build on commitment and perseverance in achieving a terrific goal. For those with unstructured lives and less discipline, the marathon offers a sense of camaraderie and positive peer pressure to get them swept up in the excitement of racing."

Review your past races. Olympic marathoner and coach Benji Durden, one of the most prolific and successful marathoners of the late 1970s, visited Scott Pengelly, PhD, noted and highly respected sport psychologist. Dr. Pengelly gave Durden some mental exercises that allowed him to review his past races and, specifically, mistakes he had made. They reviewed the mental videotape so that Durden could selectively find and correct the errors he made in prior competitions. This fine-tuning with a sports consultant was helpful and a step that Durden recommends for all competitive athletes.

Set specific goals. Kardong believes that at every level of the sport, whether you are a college athlete, an elite Olympian, a masters runner, or a weekend warrior, all of us can learn a great deal from our mental training regimens. He recommends setting goals for a race. But also break the race down into quarters, then set benchmarks for each of the quarters and expect certain feelings, emotions, and twinges to occur at all stages. Anticipate as much as possible both the good feelings and maybe some unpleasantness. Expect anything and everything to happen. If you do this mental preparation, you will be so prepared for long-distance racing that the entire experience will feel as if you had been running marathons for years.

Learn the course—thoroughly. Nothing can rattle your calm or your race plan like unexpected twists or uphills on a race course. Plaatjes's intricate preparation for the World Championship course in Stuttgart included studying information that he received beforehand about the course contours and discussing it with a training partner who had run the course in

---

SECRETS OF SUCCESS: AMBY BURFOOT

After 35 years in the running business and 25 years at *Runner's World,* here are some tips from athlete and journalist Amby Burfoot.

- Not everyone is born to be a Frank Shorter, a Steve Prefontaine, a Joan Benoit Samuelson. You must set goals that are realistic.

- Pursue the purity of the sport. "My theme is to finish the marathon, not to win it or set a special record, but just to finish it," Burfoot says.

- Recognize the courage and discipline you're gaining from running. "It gave me the courage to go back to college and to get a good job," Burfoot says.

---

another competition. "You have to prepare for every condition, every detail," says Plaatjes.

Prepare for the Wall. When you train for a marathon, you are constantly aware of energy levels. Everyone hits the proverbial Wall, the point about 20 miles into a marathon when you've just about exhausted your physical and mental energy. It is a matter of degree and how you respond to the Wall that separates the winners from those in the rest of the pack. If you can visualize the Wall—that feeling of fatigue and sense of gloom and doom—before it happens, you can plan ahead and anticipate a different outcome. The Wall is just as much physical as it is emotional. Practice hitting it before you get there.

Chill out before the race. In high school, Olympic marathoner Kenny Moore suffered from extreme prerace anxiety to the point of near exhaustion. "I was practically comatose worrying about my race and the competition," he says. "My coach was great at reading the symptoms and told me to mellow out and save all that apprehension for the race. I was burning up a lot of calories just being frightened, and it was important to have a coach who could intervene with a calming effect." To calm yourself down before big events, practice breathing exercises or listen to soothing music.

Pick a positive distraction. Durden says that he can always predict when he is going to do well in a marathon race. He usually knows it is his day when he comes to the start with a wonderful feeling of positive arousal and not an overwhelming feeling of anxiety. He once found a picture of himself at a marathon race start reading a science fiction book; this was his warmup and positive distraction and arousal state. He won that day!

Build your confidence. In the Montreal Olympics in 1976, where Kardong finished fourth, he left little up to chance. "I knew the course well, so that enhanced my imagery and internal memory in my preparation," Kardong says. "I imagined the runners going out too fast and my response to that. I rehearsed my pace—slow at first and then picking it up. I practiced my breathing in all sets of circumstances. I imagined someone surging and leading the pack, and I reminded myself that I could do that . . . I had the necessary training. I think it is important to remind yourself and to build on your confidence level when you race."

Visualize your opponents. Before mental preparation was fashionable or even had a label, Kardong was doing it. "I prepared myself by imaging myself running against the big guys—the stars of marathoning," he says.

SECRETS OF SUCCESS:
MARK PLAATJES

F Is for Fatigue

Champion marathoner Mark Plaatjes has several prescriptions for success. "You need to experience the fatigue factor when you train, because inevitably, you will hit the big F when you race. Know how it feels to be wiped out," he says. "It really helps to have a full 26.2-mile training run under your belt at a comfortable pace. Not everyone can do it, but if you can, go for it."

Plaatjes notes that racing can be very strategic, and a good marathoner should try to relax mentally during the first 13 miles. "Give your mind a break during the first half, because you're going to need every ounce of mental energy for the second half of the race." Plaatjes says that marathoners should pace themselves both physically and mentally and not dig down too hard emotionally until the last part of the race.

Plaatjes, the mental marathoner, is also attuned to his own physiology. As a physical therapist in Boulder, Colorado, he knows the red flags, the warnings of overtraining and burnout. "When I start to hurt or my Achilles tendons are burning, I cut back my training; I do not push through it," he explains. "I get deep massage therapy very often, and I listen to my body and pay attention to all the signals of distress."

"In each race I saw Frank Shorter and Bill Rodgers out there, and I knew exactly what I had to do in my mind to beat them. I studied their strides, their habits, their surges, and when they seemed to be fatigued. I had a mental notebook of every component of their racing styles. I practiced racing every waking moment in my head so that I could beat the competition."

See yourself winning. Kim Jones, one of the top female marathoners in the world, has had several near wins at Boston and New York City. "There are always two women runners who beat me: Olga Markova (the Russian star) and Wanda Panfil, a terrific competitor from Poland. I know they are the ones to beat, because they show up at the big races and beat me in the last few miles. I have my homework assignment this year, and that is to practice visualizing both of them on the course and surging on them, out-kicking them, and beating them!" Jones has done very well on her homework. Her career reads like the *Guinness Book of World Records*. She has had 17 races at 2:33 or faster, and she ran a personal record (PR) of 2:26:40 in Boston in 1991.

Anticipate the letdown. Durden knew exactly what it would take to beat the best. He had to believe in himself and have supreme confidence in his training. But he also knew that running a marathon is tough. "I had to plan in advance to not feel great all the time," he says. "In my mental preparation it was important for me to know that at some point in the 26.2-mile race, I was not going to be on top of the world. So I anticipated a letdown, some pain, and lots of fatigue. Then I anticipated a coping strategy. I used a mantra—a few words to get me back to a mental and competitive toughness. I always said, 'I'm okay, I'm all right, and I'm doing fine.'"

Build a bubble for yourself. In one race, Jones tangled with two Japanese runners who threw water on her feet during an aid stop at the 18-mile point. "I really lost it with these women. They wanted to wet my shoes down so that I would blister and have to slow up," she says. "It's a trick that is often used to upset competitors. It really got to me; I was enraged, screaming obscenities at them and, of course, using up valuable energy with all my rage." This episode was an important experience for Jones. She learned that no matter what happens out there, you must stay focused, completely within yourself, and not allow any distractions to pierce your concentration. She now goes out to a race emotionally charged with positive energy. Metaphorically, she surrounds herself with an invisible bubble that allows her to be insulated from the chaos and the behavior of other athletes. "I now know that I can't let stuff get to me; I must remain cool and calm and run my own race. I now know that I have to take responsibility for my surges and my relaxation periods and not get caught up in the emotions of the crowd. I have to maintain focus at all times."

Be prepared for exhaustion. Durden has a formula for dealing with the inevitable fatigue and pain that occur in the marathon. "I practice losing control in my mental preparation so that at mile 18 or 20, when I go into glycogen depletion and hit the Wall, I know how to respond," he says. "I remind myself that this feeling of total exhaustion is inevitable and not to give in. I tell myself to relax, not to panic, even though I'm losing control.

It is truly a mind game at this point. And if you can expect the unexpected, you can emotionally lick anyone. Once, in a race, my fatigue was so overwhelming that I forgot my mantra, so I just made up stuff as I went along."

Go easy on yourself. "If you are competing and expecting great results in every race, you are bound to set yourself up for failure," says Durden. "Know that it is okay to make mistakes. If your shoes are too tight or you are not getting enough fluid replacement, stop and check in with yourself. Have confidence in your racing ability. A marathon is a long, long, strategic race. There is a margin for error. Good marathoners can stop, stretch their muscles, and then get back in and win a race.

Relax while you visualize. When the weather is bad and Jones's asthma is flaring, she will do 3 hours on her treadmill instead of running on the road. "I try and relax when I train so that I will take this muscle memory with me to the race," she says. "Then I will visualize all the surroundings: the environment, the hills, and the topography of the race. I will continue to relax throughout these visualizations. I will ride that fine line in my imagery of being focused yet relaxed, working on a solid pace yet not straining, and seeing the competition without having a panic attack. In my imagery I always catch Wanda Panfil and Olga Markova, and I always see

SECRETS OF SUCCESS:
DON KARDONG

A Race to Grow Into

Olympic marathoner Don Kardong believes that no youngster should ever run a marathon—and many experts believe that athletes should not run marathons until after they have stopped growing, perhaps even after college. "This gives you a chance to develop some sound speed strategies from 5-K and 10-K distances," he says. "There is a certain maturity that comes with the marathon; older athletes seem to cope and respond better to this distance. Emotionally and psychologically, the marathon is a better fit for someone who is over 25, because we tend to know ourselves better by then."

myself out-kicking them. The trick now is to bring this visual to the real world, to the big race."

Keep a healthy perspective. Jones has a healthy outlook on life. After she suffered a major asthma attack in the 1992 New York City Marathon and had to be raced to a hospital in an ambulance, she realized that this marathon business could be dangerous, even fatal, for her. She started reevaluating her goals and decided to loosen up a bit with her training and road racing. Now when she races, she notices things as trivial as the shoes of the reporters in the lead car on a marathon course.

Make your imagery come true. Kardong is a student and practitioner of imagery and visualization strategies. He is emphatic about certain races where he prepared his imagery religiously. He knows that his most successful competitions were after a complete mental rehearsal for weeks in advance, such as one race in Carlsbad, California. "I desperately wanted to win," says Kardong. "Frank Shorter was going to race, and I needed to beat him; it was very important to me. So for weeks in advance, I visualized the course, the weather, the spectators, the whole scene. I even saw Shorter vividly in my imagery. I practiced surging and out-kicking Shorter; each time it became easier for me. Finally, on race day, everything I had imaged was there, including Shorter. Sure enough, I surged and beat him, and it seemed perfectly natural since I had done it in my mind's eye so many times in the prior weeks."

Give yourself some time off. Jones has a unique strategy for recovery after a hard race: She takes 4 weeks off after a major marathon. She believes that the mind, body, and soul need a major respite, a time-out from the harshness and pounding of road racing. "I just kick back for a whole month, eat a lot of chocolate, gain some weight, and take care of my emotional and physical needs," she says. "This is my freshening-up period. I believe that the body needs to go back to baseline in order to achieve another peak training period."

THE BENEFITS OF A GOOD COACH

Moore, a writer for *Sports Illustrated*, lives constantly with the images and metaphors of his former high school coach and mentor, the late Bob Newland Sr. "I think more than any other single component in running, a good coach is where the training and understanding of strategy begins," Moore says. "Even today as I get older and wiser, I am still examining the

SECRETS OF SUCCESS:
BENJI DURDEN

Mental Pacing from One Who Knows

Benji Durden, a coach with a 2:09:58 marathon PR (personal record), offers this three-stage approach to marathon racing.

Stage 1: This is the warmup, the first 10 miles of the 26.2-mile race. Durden tries to run the race at a leisurely pace, usually 10 seconds slower than optimal speed. For him, that's a 5:02 mile. He tries to talk to other runners, engaging them in dialogue and observing the scenery on the race course. He can tell immediately who is too tight and who is struggling by the way other athletes respond to him. It is usually the relaxed ones who will talk, and those are the ones whom he will see at the finish in the top five.

Stage 2: This is the second 10 miles, the "quiet down and get serious" racing mode. Here Durden gets introspective and prepares himself for the serious part of the race. This is where he lets go of the internal process. This is the quiet, "check-in-with-the-body" time. Here he may check out who the leaders are.

Stage 3: Finally, the last 6.2 miles. This is the actual race for Durden. He mentally rehearses this part all the time. The race is no longer a marathon at this point, but a rough-and-tumble 10-K race. Intensity is high during the third stage; pain is there but is deflected away from body and mind. This is where he intimidates his competitors and inflicts as much psychological damage as possible on the others by surging and creating a lot of tension in the remaining athletes. Or, if he is way ahead of the pack, Durden reverts to the tactics of stage one and starts chatting with the people in the lead car of spectators. He also allows himself to take in the scenery and enjoy the weather.

relationship between mind and body. For me, the physiology part is very important, but what seems to supersede that is having a coach who knows you, understands you, and can set limits for your training needs."

As coach, Newland was adept at knowing the talent of his athletes. He could best understand athletes by knowing their backgrounds, situations at home, girlfriends or boyfriends, and general pressures from their schools and families. Having a coach with such keen sensitivity to one's personality was quite rare, says Moore. "Mr. Newland knew who you were," he says. "Instead of dictating a set of mental practice strategies to improve your running, he would say, '*This* is what I see in you, and this is why I'm going to suggest a particular workout.' He would individualize every situation and take each athlete into account based on his own assessment of them as people as well as physical specimens. His approach was very rational, and he gave each person the ability to manage his own psychological and physiological resources."

Moore learned more lessons in management after high school. He went to the University of Oregon in Eugene and became a student of the famed Olympic track and field coaching czar, the late Bill Bowerman. Under Bowerman, Moore had to learn some tough lessons. Being a compulsive overachiever, Moore was always getting hurt and falling apart from overtraining. Bowerman told him to cut back on mileage and move to a more responsible training schedule of light days mixed with some heavier workouts, as opposed to pushing hard on every training run. "At one point, after I'd been sick a lot, Bowerman took me aside," says Moore. "He told me that for 3 weeks he would give me a workout schedule that included cross-training in the pool, weights, and a very specific regimen of lower training mileage. Intellectually, I knew where my coach was coming from, but emotionally, it wasn't getting through.

"Toward the end of his 3-week experiment, my times improved dramatically, even though I thought I wasn't working very hard. My point is that sometimes marathon athletes need help in assessing their goals in relationship to their work ethic and the type of physiology they have. Often more mileage is not better mileage. In fact, in my case, my work ethic was so strong that it was destroying me as a marathon athlete. I was fortunate to have a coach who could diagnose and correct the problem."

Forty years later, Moore says that his two coaches were instrumental in releasing him from some bad habits and patterns that ultimately might have been very destructive. "I think about my leaving Stanford Law School and beginning a career as a journalist. My coaches gave me the strength and insight to make those tough decisions, go against the grain, and tell my parents that I wasn't going to be a lawyer. Those are tough decisions to make and even harder to fulfill, but I had some very powerful mentors as an athlete."

WORKSHEET: MENTAL TRAINING
FOR MARATHONING

Review these mental training techniques before your next training run. You'll want to customize these tools to meet your own goals and needs and take note of what images or techniques work best for you.

Use affirmations and self-talk. Practice these during training as well as racing. Tell yourself during a tough race or workout, "I can do this; I can tough it out." Don't let negative thoughts such as "I'm tiring" or "I don't think I can out-kick this racer" creep in. If you stumble or another runner elbows you, tell yourself, "Stay calm; get back on pace." Choose a cue word or phrase such as "Steady" or "Keep your pace" to use during tough spots during the race.

Breathe right. Practice full breathing regularly (see Chapter 4 for specific practice steps). Before your race, you may want to listen to a specific piece of music to practice relaxed, comfortable breathing. You may want to pair an image, such as crossing the finish line of the race, with your breathing routine.

Meditate. Meditation during a race or training will help you shut out the outside world and concentrate on your own race. You might choose a mantra such as Durden's "I'm okay, I'm all right, and I'm doing fine" to repeat before and during the race to help you concentrate and stay relaxed.

Relax. After hard workouts, practice progressive relaxation to relax your muscles. Establish your own relaxation routine with an audiotape. Practice a mini relaxation session, perhaps using deep breaths or counting backward from 10 to calm yourself or relax overly tense muscles, say, in your neck. Practice relaxing during workouts so you can call up the relaxation response during races if needed.

Practice imagery and visualization. To begin guided imagery, identify how you view images by filling out the questionnaire on page 56. For im-

SECRETS OF SUCCESS:
KENNY MOORE

Know When to Back Off

Newcomers should take it easy on their first couple of long runs, advises two-time Olympian Kenny Moore. "Get comfortable racing on the track, do many 10-K races, get pushed a bit in the pack, and know and experience that congestion," he suggests. "Going into a big race, you have to have a race plan; you have to know where you expect to be at certain splits. And don't worry about anyone else. Run your own race. If you keep getting injured, then you better pay close attention to your physiology." Listen to your body, he advises. "Take pride in knowing that if you kick back and have some relaxed days, you will improve your racing and better your PR (personal record)."

agery practice, watch film clips of the Boston Marathon, the New York City Marathon, or other major races. (You can order these through ads in sports magazines.) You'll find a guided imagery program on page 240.

Consider your opponents. Durden embraces the notion that you have to know who the competition is. You should visualize yourself racing, visualize all the runners in the race, and visualize yourself finishing and winning. He admonishes the athletes he coaches to break down each component: the physical and the emotional as well as the other athlete. Durden says that if you can't visualize the other athletes in the field and know in your gut what they can do out there, then you haven't prepared adequately.

Visualize technique. In your mind, watch yourself running a marathon, slow down your visualization, and correct any mistakes you see. Study your form and style throughout the race and work on improving your pack running, hill climbing, or whatever areas of your technique need improvement. Practice mentally first and then incorporate those changes on the road.

Build a victory image. Nearly every marathon image we have comes from a televised image of an Olympic gold medalist coming across in record

┌───┐

SECRETS OF SUCCESS:
CHRISTINE CLARK

Time management is as important a mental skill as any other you could bring to competitive athletics. And no one knows this more than Christine Clark, MD, pathologist at the Providence Medical Center in Anchorage, Alaska, mother of two, and Olympic marathoner.

"I try and keep life simple; my husband and I both try and keep a nice balance in our life, kids, work, running, and the pleasures of outdoor life," she says.

Here are Dr. Clark's tips for balancing life and your sport.

- Learn to juggle or multitask so that you can get lots done and have time for training.

- Build a support system around you, including spouse, family, and friends.

- Send laundry to the cleaners if you're stressed.

- Work on self-motivation. "There are days that I'm just dead tired from work, and I just know I have to get my training miles in, so I just remind myself how good it will feel once I get going," Clark says.

└───┘

time, aching, completely fatigued, and on the edge of collapse. It is great to win, but reframe those images of yourself as well trained, well conditioned, and coming across the tape after 26.2 arduous miles with a smile, a sense of accomplishment, and having energy to spare.

Use visual motor behavior rehearsal (VMBR). Visualize yourself in a marathon; focus on enhancing your technique and analyzing and mentally correcting errors. If you tend to start too fast, practice watching yourself starting and maintaining a steady, reasonable pace. If you run poorly in a pack, watch your behavior to figure out what you can do to smooth out your pack running and mentally practice those changes. While training, practice the corrected behavior. Before races, imagine all the details of the race and how you will meet challenges that might arise. Practice switching back and forth between a relaxed phase and a ready-to-win state of mind (see page 65 for specific steps).

Have a prerace routine. Anticipate, prepare for, and minimize as many distractions as possible. At the race site, check out the surroundings, the noise of the crowd, and the weather. Like any outdoor sport, marathoning is affected by heat, humidity, a wet course, and wind. Take it all in and accept it. Look around to see who your competitors are. Thirty minutes before race time, move into your PTEZ, or perfect timing and energy zone. Practice relaxed breathing; visualize yourself running the course, passing significant mile marks, taking fluids, dealing with adversity, and finishing strongly. Tell yourself that you will do well in this race. Do any prerace rituals that make you more comfortable, such as double-knotting your shoelaces. Jones looks around the starting line to see who is there and then tries to forget about who is and who isn't competing. She then sets her mind to running her own race. Now you are ready.

CHAPTER 15

Mountain Biking: Convert Fear into Power and Precision

Mountain biking tends to bring out the wild side in people, especially those who are looking for a new adventure. "The sport has emerged in a decade and a half as a major recreational pastime as well as a very competitive event," says Nelson Pena, former executive editor of *Mountain Bike* magazine and a rider who has followed the sport carefully since its inception. "We see athletes who have blown out knees from downhill skiing who are now ready for more adrenaline rushes. Mountain biking may be analogous to surfing: Those who take up the sport as racers are a breed apart."

This sport has come a long way since its inception in 1982. A little more than 2 decades later, there are more than 765 models of mountain bikes and about 9 million mountain bike enthusiasts (and the numbers continue to grow). Approximately 30,000 of those race on weekends, some seriously but some just for fun. "It is a bit like the 10-K fun run," says Pena. "There are hotshots who run a 5-minute mile up in the front, but there is the over-9-minute-per-mile crowd that is part of the pack as well."

The National Off-Road Bike Association (NORBA) circuit has dozens of races throughout the United States each year, with downhill and cross-country events.

Some of the bigger races in the United States are now televised. The notorious downhill mountain bike event of the year is the Kamikaze Race at Mammoth Mountain in northern California, known as the Eliminator. Some races attract as many as 10,000 spectators, including some big-name sponsors who pay handsome prize money. In fact, the International Olympic Committee created an Olympic venue for cross-country mountain bike competition beginning at the 1996 Atlanta Olympic Games.

But even if you have no interest in racing, mountain biking can be a challenging sport. In this chapter you'll find tips from experts that can help you improve your riding skills, whether for racing or just for making tough climbs or descents.

BEFORE YOU HIT THE TRAILS

Mental training plays a crucial role in mountain biking, whether a recreational outing on an easy trail or a screaming downhill in elite competition. It can help you improve your abilities and harness your fear; you can learn to improve your riding by thinking positively and visualizing successful runs. Here's how some of the experts do it.

Analyze your abilities. One key to success is to passively analyze your mental and physical abilities. World-class mountain bike racer Paul Thomasberg believes that if you don't actively think about your skills, but allow them to work passively, you will learn new skills more efficiently. "You have to ride in that split-second motion of time and space," he says.

Learn to react quickly. In sports such as skiing and mountain biking, says Thomasberg, the key is adjusting to a situation and adjusting very quickly. "It is all about hand-eye coordination and being very relaxed when you start to fly down the course," he says.

Practice, practice, practice. World-class mountain bike racer Mike King is not only a champion on the course but also one who really studies the subtleties of biking. "I watch a lot of video; I observe form and substance," he says. "I'm a smooth rider and am very technical with my racing style. I do a lot of visualization in the privacy of my hotel room. I memorize the course, the terrain, the environment, and everything that I might interact with. My worst nightmare is to not have enough mental practice time in advance."

Build in some time off. Some athletes get carried away and overtrain to try to build excitement in their regimens. "It is a big mistake," says King.

"Don't overtrain; it will lead to overkill and performance decrement. Sometimes young riders get caught up in the adrenaline rush and do too much training. Don't do it; you need recovery time."

Visualize your whole day. Before each race, Thomasberg writes out a visualization script that covers every aspect of his day. "I write down what I do from the moment I wake until the moment of the race start," he ex-

MENTAL MASTERS

Alison Dunlap competed in her second Olympics in 2000, in Sydney, but her first in mountain biking. She competed at the 1996 Atlanta Games in road cycling.

Tinker Juarez is a two-time Olympian who started racing in 1986 in the inner city of Los Angeles. He is a three-time national cross-country champ, ranked 36th in the world, and won a gold medal at the 1995 Pan Am Games. He started as a BMX racer and then moved to mountain biking.

Mike King won the 1993 Mountain Bike Downhill World Championships and the Dual Slalom National Championships in France. Before 1992, he was a BMX racer.

Nelson Pena is former executive editor of *Mountain Bike* magazine and an avid mountain biker.

Paul Thomasberg, from Bend, Oregon, was the 1993 bronze medalist at the Mountain Bike Downhill World Championships in Durango, Colorado, and placed fourth in the cross-country at the same championships. In 1976, he qualified for the youth Olympic training team in downhill skiing.

John Tomac is a great mountain bike racer, in cross-country as well as downhill. He won the 1991 World Championship in the cross-country, has won the famous Mammoth Mountain Downhill in California, and was the 1991 national champion in downhill. He also won the US cross-country title in 1996 and the US downhill in 1997.

plains. "I chart my eating, my rituals . . . every detail. I visualize the tuning up of my bike and putting my race numbers on. I visualize the setting up of my equipment, my warmup, and my breathing. I visualize every part so carefully that when I get to the start, I'm already relaxed from the mental rehearsal."

Stay focused. In mountain biking, the athlete must concentrate on the sport to be proficient and to avoid injury. "I'm married, have two kids, and a house payment to make," says Thomasberg. "If I'm worried about a sick child or paying bills, my riding is out of focus; I'm not in flow. And yet, if you stay focused, the benefits, including financial, are terrific. A good racer can make six figures racing the circuit."

Memorize that course. Top mountain bike racer John Tomac is clear about one thing. You have to have a comprehensive visual and kinesthetic memory bank that locks in the corners, the turns, and every contour of the downhill course. During his six to eight preruns, Tomac gets a feel, or a kinesthetic sense, of the course. He does not study maps or pictures, but goes to the course way before the race to warm up. From the time that he finishes the warmup till the moment of the race, he's on autopilot. "When you know that you are about to hit a 6-mile course for 12 minutes and reach speeds of 60 miles per hour, you'd better have a good visual sense of where you are going," he says. "Split-second timing doesn't count; you have to feel every motion in anticipation of the next motion."

Mentally rehearse. Tomac prepares meticulously for each race. "I need to review the course many times over so that it becomes a part of my visual memory. I need to rehearse each corner so that I know how I am going to negotiate a turn." There are certain courses in downhill that have a 30 percent grade, he points out, and on a hill that steep, one small mistake could be dangerous. One course that Tomac loves to negotiate is on Mount Snow in Vermont. "It has a lot of variables—open slopes, hidden terrain—you see the rocks and then you don't see them," he says. "The roots get slick, and you have to prepare to hit the racing line with absolute finesse or you wipe out. Corners are either negotiated by entering from the outside with an exit to the inside or vice versa. But this decision is made well in advance: It's part of your prerace visualization strategy."

Visualize the race in advance. "I go to bed every night and visualize a course," says King. "I practice imagery on the chairlift, and I am always preparing myself. I run through the whole course in detail. I rehearse which racing lines to take on the hill and how to maneuver certain turns. I always decide in advance which line I will take going into a curve. I never leave anything to chance. It is always predetermined in my visualization workout. You have to be a student of concentration and focus in this sport. You have to visualize all aspects of a race and not worry about anybody else."

Allow your setbacks to motivate you. In 2003, reigning female World Cup Champion Alison Dunlap crashed hard on a high-speed descent and violently separated her shoulder. Dunlap had about a minute lead when her hand slipped off her handlebars and she went down. She underwent surgery that August and has been working on coming back ever since.

Instead of seeing her injury as a setback, Dunlap has focused on viewing it in a healthy way by respecting the fact that athletes often are injured, by knowing that trying to come back too fast can be detrimental to her overall career, and by using the injury as an opportunity to enhance her mental training. "Injury is motivating; it is a whole new level of energy," she says. "I'm focused on coming back with a vengeance; I can take this time to visualize and plan my goals."

OVERCOME FEARS

The following tips can help you get control of your race or a challenging ride.

Stifle negative thoughts. "I get nervous about certain things—the unexpected, the unavoidable events," says Thomasberg. "I get terribly anxious coming down a mountain and thinking about a front-end failure, a blowout, and inevitable crash. If you think about all the potential dangers, you can get yourself very frightened."

Harness your fears. Thomasberg likes to take that anxious, fearful energy and harness it into something productive, such as racing his bike at 55 miles per hour down a treacherous mountain. He often practices a course in his mind, visualizing the turns, corners, and soft spots of the mountain and getting butterflies in his stomach just by imagining the race. Then he channels any free-floating anxiety into a productive focus on race preparation. He likes to take the emotion of fear and convert it to positive energy. "In mountain biking, there is a lot of danger, and if you let the fear overcome you, you are going to have an unpleasant experience. I like to acknowledge the fear, channel it, and refocus it toward a positive energy state."

SECRETS OF SUCCESS:
JOHN TOMAC

You Don't Have to Race

Top mountain bike racer John Tomac, who won the famed Mammoth Mountain Downhill in California, advises:

- Do adequate preparation to decrease anxiety and enhance internal focus. Do your homework.

- Don't expect to get much out of your racing if you haven't done your training, both physically and mentally.

- If you find yourself stressing out over racing, says Tomac, forget about racing. Just enjoy the recreational side of mountain biking.

Don't overanalyze. "Zen and the art of mountain biking" would be a good theme for Thomasberg and his style of riding. For that matter, it fits his entire lifestyle. "You want to passively analyze your skills, not overanalyze them and not overly prepare when riding a mountain bike. There is so much delicate timing here that it's important to mentally rehearse a great deal of your hills and racing strategies. You want to prepare for a race, but don't overdo it; allow yourself to be spontaneous with good reaction time and a feeling of confidence that you can handle any unexpected problem."

Think of yourself as part of the bike. When all the pieces come together, Thomasberg is one with his bike. A great ride is like a meditation, he says. "There is nothing in my mind except the moment, the trail, the mountains, my reflexes, and my bike. We are all in a space of oneness."

Do a last-minute mental rehearsal. King notes that the key to great racing is to start off slowly when you practice and get a feel from the practice runs. Do five runs at all-out full speed. Then go back and mentally rehearse what you just did on the course and make any corrections on your visual rehearsal screen as necessary. He also reminds riders to listen to their bodies and to not overdo it.

Think positively. To stay focused and away from strange thoughts and distractions that can lead to problems, world-ranked mountain bike racer Tinker Juarez doesn't allow himself to think negatively. "When you race, you cannot think about strange falls or crashes. You cannot allow yourself the imagery of 'what happens if I crash?'"

Talk yourself out of tenseness. King talks to himself during races. "I always say, 'Hey, take it easy; don't overcorrect; go easy on the turns.' I remind myself internally to take a turn here, enter there, break there, stay calm, and have fun. I constantly remind myself to stay very relaxed. I often laugh to myself because it helps take the edge off the tension. I ride better when I'm not tense."

Stick to your game plan. King knows an obstacle or a bump when he sees it, because he has already mentally rehearsed the object and his reaction to it. He knows in advance how to handle the rough spots, the jumps, and downhill speed. He has total confidence in his skills and doesn't force himself to go over the edge.

Keep your cool. Injury is something that crosses King's mind, but only for a nanosecond of time. "You don't want to think about the negatives, because if you start focusing on injury, your days are numbered," he says. "Remember to stay focused, believe in yourself, and maintain calmness when you race. If you can incorporate all of these things, the fear will convert to adrenaline, and that conversion will lead to a good mental attitude." If he were ever to have concern, it would be about having a mechanical failure at 60 miles per hour on a turn, going over the bars, and getting wiped out. But he quickly erases any of those thoughts and reminds himself that he has tested his equipment, has a great mechanic, and has supreme confidence in himself.

WORKSHEET: MENTAL TRAINING
FOR MOUNTAIN BIKING

Review these mental training techniques before your next mountain bike ride or race. You'll want to customize this program to meet your own goals and needs and take note of what images or techniques work best for you.

Use affirmations and self-talk. Practice these during training as well as racing. Tell yourself during a tough race or training ride, "I can do this;

SECRETS OF SUCCESS:
PAUL THOMASBERG

Three Steps to Better Biking

Paul Thomasberg is a mountain bike racer who lives and breathes the sport. He lives in Bend, Oregon, one of the most beautiful mountain landscapes in America, and gets to practice his craft in some very high places.

Thomasberg likes to get his heart rate to maximum level. He gets uncomfortable when he is not taking risks or racing; he knows no fear. He got his first taste of speed racing and falling with the forces of gravity as a downhill skier qualifying for the youth Olympic training team in 1976.

He races 20 events a year, including two tours of Europe. He cross-trains with skiing to stay in shape. He also rides his stationary bike for 40 minutes every morning before breakfast. When he trains, he rides his bike 3 to 4 hours a day, 5 days a week.

Thomasberg subscribes to the school of mind-body togetherness and has a three-stage program for training. His program is the following:

- Relaxation. As you race a steep hill, try to loosen up. By relaxing, you will be able to absorb bumps better, and your reaction time will be faster. If you lose control during a downhill, you will be able to recover faster.

- Confidence. Confidence is paramount to good racing. The way to gain confidence is to ride in control. Stay on that thin line of control, occasionally crossing it to test yourself, but don't get too far over it.

- Concentration. Learning new skills and going faster on a mountain bike requires 110 percent concentration. If you have something on your mind, you will be distracted and have serious problems.

If you lose relaxation, you will hit bumps harder and slow reaction time, warns Thomasberg. If you don't have confidence, you might hit your brakes too early. If you lose concentration, you won't be able to read the trail as well, and you could lose control of your bike.

I can make this corner." Don't allow negative thoughts such as "I'm not gonna make this turn" or "I don't think I can make up the time I need." If you fall, tell yourself, "Stay calm; put it behind you." Choose a cue word or phrase such as "You can do it" to use in tough spots during the race.

Breathe right. Practice full breathing regularly (see Chapter 4 for specific practice steps). Before your race, you may want to listen to a specific piece of music to practice relaxed, comfortable breathing. You might pair an image, such as crossing the finish line of a race or seeing yourself climbing powerfully, with your breathing routine.

Meditate. Meditation during a race or training will help you shut out the outside world and concentrate on your own race. You might choose a mantra such as King's "Take it easy; don't overcorrect; go easy on the turns" to repeat before and during the race to help you concentrate and stay relaxed.

Relax. After hard workouts, practice progressive relaxation to relax your muscles. Establish your own relaxation routine with an audiotape. Practice a mini relaxation session, perhaps using deep breaths or counting backward from 10 to calm yourself or relax a tense muscle. Practice relaxing during rides so you can call up the relaxation response to calm yourself, if needed. If you're about to begin a particularly tricky, steep descent in a race or on a ride, for instance, you may want to relax tense muscles so you can concentrate fully on successfully finishing the course.

Practice imagery and visualization. To begin guided imagery, identify how you view images by filling out the questionnaire on page 56. For imagery practice, videotape actual races or record races shown on television and watch those. You'll find a guided imagery program on page 240.

Consider your opponents. Opponents in mountain bike races may cause problems, especially in tight turns on steep slopes. Thomasberg tries to visualize who will be out there at the precise moment when he takes a turn, thus reducing his risk by preparing mentally for each turn on each downhill.

Visualize technique. Certainly for mountain bikers, the fear of the course and wiping out on a big hill can be overwhelming. In your mind, watch yourself racing, cornering, and descending, and slow down your visualization and correct any mistakes you see. Go to extremes when practicing your imagery. Take yourself to the edge by feeling the fear, then come back into your mental picture by experiencing the joy and exhilaration of riding and cruising at high speed. Practice both.

Build a victory image. Mountain biking can be dangerous, especially on the Mammoth Mountain Eliminator. This is a straight shot down from 10,000 feet at lightning speed on a crusty, rock-filled course. Just thinking about this descent can engender some anxiety and fear. Mentally rehearse the course with no rocks, no slides, and solid tracks for your tires. Take a moment and enjoy your last 100 yards at warp speed with no falls, no slips, and no crashes. You can do it; you just have to rehearse the correct picture.

Use visual motor behavior rehearsal (VMBR). Visualize yourself in a race; focus on enhancing your technique and analyzing and mentally correcting errors. While training, practice the corrected behavior. Before races, imagine all the details of the race and how you will meet challenges that might arise. Practice switching back and forth between a relaxed phase and a ready-to-win state of mind (see page 65 for specific steps). If you're not racing, but just riding, you can still benefit from these techniques. Before a tough climb or descent, imagine the obstacles you'll encounter—a slippery corner, a log to jump, a steep slope—and visualize how you will successfully get past them.

Have a prerace routine. Anticipate, prepare for, and minimize as many distractions as possible. At the race site, check out the surroundings, the crowd, the weather, and the noise. Is it cloudy? Sunny? Drizzly? Register these factors. Look around to see who your competitors are. Thirty minutes before race time, move into your PTEZ, or perfect timing and energy zone. Block out the past and the future and focus on the now. Practice relaxed breathing; visualize yourself riding the course, dealing with roots, rocks, gravel, or mud and finishing strongly. Tell yourself that you will ride as well as you ever have before. Do any prerace rituals that make you more comfortable—checking your brakes and quick release skewers, and so on. Even if you're not racing, these same tips will work before you begin a challenging or intimidating ride.

CHAPTER 16

Running on Road and Track: Optimize Your Performance

Jeff Atkinson, a 1988 Olympic gold medalist in the 1500 meters, has said that mental preparation is the only way to completely train for a race. "My win in the Olympic Trials was marked by a steady and extensive buildup of all aspects of my training—physical as well as mental preparation. I knew my race tactics and what my strategy would be. Those pieces came together in such a way that by the time I got to the start of the race, I was certain everything would be in flow." Most athletes attribute much of their success and winning attitudes to their mental preparation and visualization strategies.

Diane Palmason, a top masters runner, coaches many 10-K runners and focuses on mental preparation. "I tell my athletes to initially prepare for the 10-K by sitting down and visualizing the entire race before they run," she says. "I tell them, 'Today you're going to do your training in your chair. Get rid of the distractions. Play the event in your head and do a lot of visualization around positive thinking and positive arousal.' I tell the athletes that they have to prepare for all the excitement, all the energy, and all the appropriate arousal energy."

The proper strategies for peak performance take time to learn and require some practice. The good news is that the more you practice, the easier these techniques become to implement in your training regimen.

GETTING READY TO MOVE

Mac Wilkins, gold-medal winner in the discus throw in the 1976 Montreal Olympics, is fond of saying, "Basically, it boils down to the fact that if you are trying to accomplish a goal on the track, and you can't visualize it, then it's pure chance if you perform well. If you visualize that goal and really see yourself performing well, however, then you have a clear target to aim for and a very high probability of achieving that success." So how does one prepare mentally, arranging all the images in place before a race on the track or on the road?

Set goals in advance. Palmason sets goals in her head days before her big races. She knows the clock, the pace, and how she should feel. "I always see myself going through every aspect of my race, from the start, to running in a crowd, to the kick, and then the finish. It is always planned way in advance. Regardless of the event, from the 800 meters to the marathon, every component is broken down in my mental rehearsal."

Enjoy your training. "One of my secrets for getting my mileage up in training and practice is to have fun and not stress out," says Palmason. "I set out to enjoy a long training run. I pick a fun place where there are birds, water, and lovely conditions so that I can enjoy the whole experience."

Visualize the perfect race. The late Olympic hurdler Willie Davenport, who had more than 20 years of competitive experience as an elite athlete, suggested that you have a vision of the perfect race before you even start your event. "Regardless of my race strategy, the most important technique gets practiced long before I enter the competition," he told me before his death. You have to prepare this vision long before the start. Davenport used to tell high school and college hotshots that they must begin each day mentally rehearsing an explosive start, the well-balanced body tension, the ideal kick, and the perfect finish. "If you don't have the mental strategies in place, you are in big trouble."

Learn to relax. Four-time Olympic 800-meter champion Maria Mutola says that athletes must gauge each event and each performance based on their levels of confidence from prior races. Each race builds in a new sense of self-esteem, a new set of goals, and a feeling of relaxed well-being. "If I can't go into a race relaxed, then I'm in trouble. I need to get to that comfortable place in my prayers, in my imagery, where I feel that all of the tension and anxiety is behind me."

Take quiet time before racing. Mutola has a prescription for athletes: Stay focused and don't get distracted by your friends, the crowd, or the social networks. "I go to these high school meets, and I see these talented athletes 2 hours before a big race expending lots of energy on socializing. They are running here and there and getting caught up with their friends, using up a lot of precious energy in the process. I suggest that all young runners find a quiet place or a quiet friend and spend some quiet time preparing for their races. It's a sacrifice for some youngsters, but we all need that emotional fine-tuning right before competition."

Think positively. Harvey Glance, three-time Olympic sprint champion and head track and field coach at the University of Alabama, writes confidence-building notes to his athletes, reminding them to think positively during their daily workouts. He says this helps them bring positive images to their races.

MENTAL MASTERS

Jeff Atkinson placed 10th in the 1500 meters in the 1988 Seoul Olympics.

Willie Davenport, who died in 2002, competed in the Olympics four times as a hurdler and once as a bobsledder.

Harvey Glance is in his sixth season as head track and field coach at the University of Alabama. He is a three-time Olympic sprint champion and won gold in the 4x100 relay in 1984.

Hal Higdon was the first American finisher at the Boston Marathon in 1964 and coaches all age levels of runners. In 1981, he won the World Veterans' Championships. He writes for *Runner's World* magazine and has written several books on running.

Maria Mutola, a four-time Olympian, won the 800 meters in the 1993 World Championship in Stuttgart, Germany, in a blistering 1:55:44 pace. She won bronze at the 1996 Olympics in Atlanta and then won gold in Sydney. In August 2003, she was awarded a check for $1 million for her gold in the IAAF Grand Prix in Belgium, the highest payday for any track and field woman ever.

Listen to your coach. Track Olympian PattiSue Plumer's strategy for competing is to know herself and her form. "A lot of times your coach, who knows you well, can see things before you do," she says. "A coach can tell you that your legs are falling flat on the ground, your steps are heavy, or your stride is a little bit too short. She can tell you that you're not leaning forward as you used to. Those are all signs of fatigue. And that is when you need to take time off and do some mental practice off the track. A good coach can pick up the cues of fatigue usually faster than you can. That's when it's time for the pool, volleyball, biking, or a variety of cross-training programs. That is when you should practice the mental side of training and give yourself a rest on the physical aspects."

See the perfect race. Most world-class track athletes, including Mutola, will tell you that when you get to the starting line, the first thing you must put in your mind is the image of the perfect race. You have to visualize an

Diane Palmason set the Canadian and world records for the 400 and 800 meters in the masters 65 to 69 age group. Her lifetime best is 2:33.4. She set a Canadian record of 1:31:40 for the half-marathon and the Canadian Marathon record of 3:14.21. She competed on the Canadian National Team in 1954 and still competes at age 65.

Mike Pigg is a top US triathlete and the number two–ranked triathlete in the world. He has won 77 out of his last 133 races from 1987 thru 1995.

PattiSue Plumer competed in the 1500 and 3000 meters in the 1988 and 1992 Olympics.

Louise Ritter is a three-time Olympian (1980, 1984, and 1988) who won the gold medal in the Olympic high jump in 1988.

Mac Wilkins is a four-time Olympian and 1976 gold medalist in the discus. He holds four world records.

explosive start, the right amount of thrust of your knees and legs, the correct tension in your lower body, the relaxed portion of your upper body, the on-target pace, the ideal kick, and the perfect finish.

THE RACE BEFORE THE RACE

Probably the best preparation for your perfect race takes place well before the actual event. Several months before the Montreal Olympic Games, in the spring of 1976, sports medicine trainers from the Soviet Union took videos and slides of the track and field stadium in downtown Montreal. They took these back home so that the Soviet athletes could study them in detail.

Many of the Soviet athletes had never competed in North America before, and the photographs allowed them to create images of themselves performing in those athletic venues. Creating these types of internal and external images (for several months in advance) served to familiarize the athletes with the competitive environment before they arrived at the Olympic Games. By reserving these images in their own memory storage, the athletes felt as if they were already at the site. Many athletes often report after prolonged imagery training a sense of déjà vu. Here's how you can prepare mentally so that unexpected conditions don't derail you during your race.

Simulate conditions. Today, taking photos or videos of foreign venues is not a state secret or even considered unusual. In fact, most coaches who have traveled internationally brief their athletes about track and road conditions many months before traveling to the venue. A wonderful example of this is Olympic gold-medal high jumper Louise Ritter, who went to great lengths to prepare for her Olympic competition in Seoul. Preparing for the trials in the spring of 1988, Ritter and her coach changed directions on her high jump approach to simulate different wind conditions in the Seoul stadium. Because the Olympics were late that year in 1988 (September and into early October), they decided to simulate weather as well. "My coach wanted me to prepare physically, mentally, and emotionally for any strange environmental situation," says Ritter. "I showed up at the track in Dallas one day, and he was flooding the high jump pit and the runway approach and hosing down everything in sight. He really wanted to eliminate any surprises in Korea that might mentally distract me from my best possible jump. We were indeed prepared for anything and everything."

Inspect the course. Many coaches will tell you that it is important to simulate the most likely conditions for any athletic venue. According to one college coach, you must learn to expect the unexpected in track competition. Nike vice president and former track and road racing star Alberto Salazar is known for his complete and absolute attention to detail when racing, including his warmup and prerace strategies. He likes to drive the entire length of a road race course to see and feel the contours, the hills, and the bumps to anticipate and prepare mentally for his quest. He leaves nothing to chance.

Memorize the route. Top US triathlete Mike Pigg believes in being meticulously prepared for each event in his races. "Once, when the race marshals led me the wrong way, I knew the course so well—I had mentally rehearsed it over and over and my confidence was so high—that I chose not to follow them," he says. "I knew they had taken a wrong turn and were leading athletes down a path of disaster. I knew my way, and I won the race."

Prepare for fatigue. For Palmason, the toughest thing to overcome in her long-distance events is fatigue, especially in the marathon and half-marathon. Left unchecked, fatigue leads to a diminished mental attitude and a desire to quit. "To counteract fatigue, I give myself permission to pause and drink water, and then I reset my pace," she says.

WINNING TIPS FOR RACE DAY

It's morning on the day of your event. Whether it's your first 5-K fun run, a grueling marathon, or the Olympic Trials, things can go wrong. Your best bet is to have an established routine.

Follow your prerace ritual. Mutola's 800-meter race preparation also includes quiet time before each competition, with a break for some music. Not just any music, but Bob Marley's "Everything's Gonna Be All Right." This gets her in the mood and in the right frame of mind. Mutola has a ritual before each race, which can vary depending on the competition and intensity of the event. "At the Barcelona Olympics, I rested, I showered, I prayed, and I listened to lots of music," she says. "Maybe I didn't do enough of each. I finished fifth in the Olympics; next time I'll rework my ritual, including a longer mental preparation strategy."

Structure your race day. Mutola literally races across the globe so that she can get more track racing experience under her belt. Like the late veteran racer

Davenport did, Mutola prepares thoroughly for each race. This includes a comprehensive mental preparation. She structures race day with a rest period (or nap, if possible) 8 hours before the competition. "Then I pray a bit before each race. In my prayers, I can see myself race. I visualize a strategy on each of my two laps for the 800 meters, and often I see my furious kick."

Know the competition. Pigg knows his competitors, but he doesn't dwell on their presence. "I'm aware of who's out there," he explains. "They're part of my memory bank, but I don't become obsessive about

SECRETS OF SUCCESS:
MIKE PIGG

Toughing It Out

Top US triathlete Mike Pigg is a road runner as well as a cyclist and a swimmer. He's been named Triathlete of the Year twice and was the second-ranked triathlete in the world when this book was written.

In triathlons, the race finishes off with the running event, so it's here where a triathlete has to make up time lost in the other events. It's also where the athlete is the most tired and prone to discouragement. Here's how Pigg recommends you get through tough runs.

- Think about your breath and your step.

- Know the course—and know it well.

- Key in on a tough competitor to push yourself just a bit harder.

- Let yourself get involved in the passion of the event.

Pigg is a firm believer in preparation—both physical and mental. "I don't chitchat before a race; I get very serious and very focused," he says. "After competing in triathlons for 11 years, I know that I have to find my zone early on, and talking usually distracts me from that zone. This is the place where I go when I'm completely mentally and psychologically fo-

them. I just know who they are, and I know some of their strengths and many of their weaknesses."

Watch the guys in back. "I always see people in back of me. I don't know how, but I can visualize these people and know exactly where they are," Davenport used to tell me. "If I'm racing out in front of other competitors, I can still see them."

Monitor your progress. Plumer has a strategy for racing that is quite different from other athletes. She does an enormous amount of mental

cused and ready to compete. This is where I go to reduce all the variables and remove any mistakes."

Pigg takes himself into his performance zone—his private quiet time— before the race begins, sometimes even the night before a big race. This is where he visits his visual imagery screen to check the water, the bike course, and the running route. Once he knows all the elements, he can build up his confidence.

Here are some triathlon tips from Pigg.

- Have your whole race day prepared in advance. Have your bike clean and all your gear ready to go.

- Lay out your equipment in the precise order that you'll need it during transitions. This is where you can make up time on other competitors.

- Know the water, the bike route, and the running course. Check out the water temperature, the road conditions, and contours and hills on the running route.

- Visualize all three elements the night before.

- Break the event down into three distinct races.

- Keep up a positive attitude throughout your training and racing.

practice both on and off the track, but when racing, she focuses on monitoring her stride, her energy level, and her stamina.

WORKSHEET: MENTAL TRAINING FOR RUNNING

Review these mental training techniques before your next run. You'll want to customize these tools to meet your own goals and needs and take note of what images or techniques work best for you.

Use affirmations and self-talk. Practice these during training as well as racing. Tell yourself during a tough race or workout, "I can do this." Don't allow negative thoughts such as "That other competitor looks fitter than I do" or "I don't think I can make up the time I need." If you have a bad start or miss a step, tell yourself, "Stay calm; put it behind you." Choose a cue word or phrase such as "You can do it" to use in tough spots during the race.

Breathe right. Practice full breathing regularly (see Chapter 4 for specific practice steps). Before your race, you may want to listen to a specific piece of music to practice relaxed, comfortable breathing. You might want to pair an image, such as crossing the finish line of the race, with your breathing routine.

Meditate. Meditation during a race or training will help you shut out the outside world and concentrate on your own race. You might choose a mantra such as "You can do it" to repeat before and during the race to help you concentrate and stay relaxed.

Relax. After hard workouts, practice progressive relaxation to relax your muscles. Establish your own relaxation routine with an audiotape. Practice a mini relaxation session, perhaps taking deep breaths or counting backward from 10 to calm yourself or relax overly tense muscles. Practice relaxing during workouts so you can call up the relaxation response during races, if needed.

Practice imagery and visualization. To begin guided imagery, identify how you view images by filling out the questionnaire on page 56. For imagery practice, watch film clips of races. You can tape race coverage from television or buy a tape on running techniques (look in sporting goods stores and in ads in running magazines). You'll find a guided imagery program on page 240.

Consider your opponents. Steve Placencia, two-time Olympian in the 10,000 meters and a fine road runner for nearly 2 decades, visualizes the

SECRETS OF SUCCESS:
HAL HIGDON

Tips to Pave Your Way

Hal Higdon, a successful road racer for many decades, also coaches at various levels of the sport. He incorporates a lot of fun with intense workouts for all competitors.

"I like to run with my high school athletes as well as my elite competitors, so I can monitor their training but also enjoy the process," he says. Road racing, for the beginner as well as for the more advanced, is all about building mental confidence and building physiological strength and conditioning.

"The mental and physical all work in synchronicity until you reach plateaus," he says. "Each new training plateau gives one a new sense of accomplishment and achievement, and then you build on that base. You are consistently building on new foundations."

Higdon always encourages building a strong aerobic base by enhancing endurance. This is accomplished by a series of daily short runs followed by a longer run every third day. At the end of your long run, try to increase your speed gently so that it builds within you a sense of confidence, strength, and conditioning. This will set the base for your next series of workouts.

Other tips from Higdon:

- Keep a daily log of your runs.

- Monitor your pulse before and after workouts.

- Stretch and warm up before runs.

- Stretch and cool down after runs.

- Keep a log of your diet.

- Note your emotional states, both highs and lows.

- Cut back your training when you feel any twinges or fatigue.

whole field. He wants to know all the credentials of everyone in the field. Then he can visualize the start, the race, the finish—and know well in advance his place in the pack and anticipate a great finish. Also, anticipate traffic jams in advance. All the great racers will tell you that the best plans for a winning race include a mental practice session, such as seeing yourself in a pack of "sardines," vulnerable to a push, a shove, and perhaps a fall. Prepare mentally for running in crowded conditions without feeling trapped.

Visualize technique. Road running is an art as well as a science. In your mind, watch yourself during a race, slow down your visualization, and correct any mistakes you see. Carefully study your style, your running form, how you start the race, and how you finish and make corrections, both in your mental image and while you're training and racing.

Build a victory image. Some of the great road races in the country— the Peachtree in Atlanta; the Falmouth on Cape Cod; the Butte to Butte in Eugene, Oregon; and the notorious Bay-to-Breakers in San Francisco— have wonderful memories and images attached to them. These are images of great competitors, wonderful costumes, outrageous outfits, and beautiful days under very blue skies. Pick your favorite race from the past, remember the feelings of exuberance and energy as you started, feel the energy of your legs and the rhythmic thumping of your heart, and remember your strong finish. This is the victory image you should take with you wherever you go for your next race.

Use visual motor behavior rehearsal (VMBR). Visualize yourself in a race; focus on enhancing your technique and analyzing and mentally correcting errors. If you lose a pace every time you grab a drink of water, practice the routine in your mind until you can do it smoothly. If you aren't giving your maximum effort during finishes, watch yourself again and again giving it your all. While training, practice the corrected behavior. Before races, imagine all the details of the race and how you will meet challenges that might arise. Imagine yourself dealing with running in a pack, coping with hot weather, a loud crowd, a misstep. Practice switching back and forth between a relaxed phase and a ready-to-win state of mind (see page 65 for specific steps).

Have a prerace routine. Anticipate, prepare for, and minimize as many distractions as possible. At the race site, check out the surroundings, the crowd, the weather, and the noise. Look around to see who your competitors are. Thirty minutes before race time, move into your PTEZ, or perfect timing and energy zone. Practice relaxed breathing. Visualize yourself running the course, surging with the leaders, leaving the pack, and finishing strongly. Tell yourself that you will do well in this race. Do any prerace rituals that make you more comfortable, such as double-knotting your shoelaces, adjusting your clothing, or jogging in place.

CHAPTER 17

Swimming and Diving: Perfect Your Performance in the Pool

Australian swimming legend Susie O'Neil has enough precious metal in her trophy case to start a small mint. Now retired, this 30-year-old has placed in just about every major event she's entered. In the 1992 Olympics in Barcelona, she won bronze in the 200-meter butterfly. At the Atlanta Olympics in 1996, she captured gold in the same event, followed by silver in the 4x100 medley, and then icing on the cake with a bronze in the 4x200 free relay. On her home court (or should I say pool) in the Sydney Olympics, O'Neil won gold in the 200-meter free, silver in the 200-meter butter, and two silvers in the 4x100 and 4x200 relays. In the midst of all that; she won a truckload of medals at the Pan Am Games, World Championships, and Commonwealth Games. She has been named Australian swimmer of the year, Australian athlete of the year, and Olympian of the year.

Along the way, mental training appears to have played a key role in O'Neil's success, using self-talk and visualization to focus.

"I did have to perpetually talk myself into believing that I was good and that I was better than everyone else who jumped into the pool," she says.

"Before race time, I always tried to relax, stay calm, rid myself of the pregame nerves, and concentrate on my game plan. On her visualization, O'Neil says: "I would place a pretend curtain up against both lanes in the pool so that I could not see anyone, no other swimmers, just see myself. I wanted to block out all the others; no distractions. I would remind myself with phrases that I was long and strong. No extra thoughts: I did not want to have any other distractions or worries that would take me away from my game plan. Very simple."

In ways, she shares the same philosophy as four-time Olympic gold medalist Janet Evans, who believes that half of everything you do is mental. When she swims, she told me: "I continue to visualize all my races days and weeks before they happen. I have never been to a competition, including the Olympic Games, where I didn't see myself win in my mental images before I got there. It is just part of the whole training package." Evans and her teammates visualize and do other mental practice sessions all season long. Sometimes they practice imagery as a whole team, but often the sessions are individual. "Whenever we are really tired from a major workout, you might find a lot of swimmers sleeping through a visualization session," she says. "But even then, the power of the mind is quite extraordinary."

STRATEGIES THAT WORK

Whether you're training for the Olympics, doing a few laps in the pool on weekends, or trying to improve your swim time in triathlons, there is much mental preparation and training you can do to improve your speed and style—not to mention how much you enjoy your workouts.

Set realistic goals. Evans and her teammates always set goals with their coach at the beginning of the season. The goals have to be realistic, both for the athlete and the coach. "Part of my mental game plan is to share with my coach what I hope to achieve throughout the year in my training. We try and set up a strategy early on. I also believe that overtraining, fatigue, and burnout are a state of mind. Certainly, we all get tired after putting in miles of laps, but the notion of burnout is really a psychological one."

Clear your mind. Your swimming workout will be a lot tougher if you bring the day's problems into the pool with you," Evans says. "I need to come to workouts with no excess baggage or preconceived notions about how I should perform. I want my workouts each day to open a new door, a new and fresh chapter, and leave the baggage behind. I want to enjoy the celebration of competition, the rhythm and dance in the water."

Take a look at your stroke. One of the best ways to help yourself visualize your stroke clearly and make needed corrections is to see yourself on videotape, says Terry Laughlin, former director of Total Immersion adult swim camps, technique specialist for the US Swimming Olympic Development Group, and fitness editor for *Swim Magazine.* "There are people who

MENTAL MASTERS

Janet Evans won four Olympic gold medals in swimming in 1988 plus a gold and silver at the 1992 Games in Barcelona. She was a member of three Olympic Teams. She also won three golds at the World Championships in 1993. She owns three world records in the 400, 800, and 1500 meters. She holds six American records, she was honored with the prestigious Sullivan award in 1989, and she has five NCAA titles. She is now on the FINA advisory panel and is working very closely with the IOC to ensure that athletes are competing clean and drug free.

Susie O'Neil competed for the Australian Olympic teams in 1992, 1996, and 2000. In Barcelona, she won bronze in the 200-meter butterfly; she won gold in the same event in Atlanta, followed by silver in the 4x100 medley and then bronze in the 4x200 free relay.

Crissy Perham was a member of the US Olympic Swim Team in Barcelona in 1992, a double gold medalist in the 400-meter freestyle and medley relays and a silver medalist in the 100-meter butterfly. Crissy is now a mom, coach, and very involved in sports management.

Terry Laughlin was director of the Total Immersion adult swim camps and is a technique specialist for the US Swimming Olympic Development Group. He formerly coached college and age-group swimmers and is fitness editor for *Swim Magazine.*

Mike Pigg was the number-two ranked triathlete in the world in 1995.

learn best visually," he says. "If you don't provide them with some sort of visual feedback or visual lesson in what you want them to do, they're always handicapped in their ability to learn." Laughlin videotapes swimmers above and below water and plays the video back in slow motion to dissect the stroke and determine what can be improved.

Trust your mentor. O'Neil places a lot of credit for her success with Scott Volkers. "He really got me to build confidence during training; he helped me to train hard, to keep my consistency in the pool, and to keep

Summer Sanders came home from her first Olympic Games in Barcelona with four medals: silver in the 200-meter individual medley, gold in the 200-meter butterfly and relay, and bronze in the 400-meter medley.

Nicole Haislett-Bacher won triple gold in the 1992 Olympics: one medal in the 200 meters, then a win in the 400 free relay, and gold in the medley relay. She finished fourth in the 100 free.

Matt Scoggins competed in the 1992 Olympic diving competition and is now the diving coach at the University of Texas at Austin. In Sydney, he was the Olympic coach and was voted NCAA coach of the year in 2002.

Kimiko Soldati won the bronze at the 2001 Goodwill Games in Australia and the silver at the World Cup that year in the 10-meter platform and has been a two-time Senior National Champion and a member of the US National Diving Team for 7 years.

Justin Dumais is the recipient of 13 national championships, five international titles, and many more honors, including third at the 2003 Pan Am Games.

Laura Wilkinson went to Sydney and brought home gold in the women's 10-meter platform. She is also the winner of the 1998 Goodwill Games dive competition, a three-time Senior National Champion in both 10-M and 3-M individual and synchro events, and the 1995 World FINA Cup bronze medalist.

motivated," she says. "As a motivation strategy, he would lay guilt on me. 'You wanna come in third, then keep doing this . . . but if you wanna win, then you need to do this.' It usually worked."

Cross-train. O'Neil says that cross-training for a swimmer is essential. Like other athletes, swimmers can enhance their focus and drive, not to mention their muscles and skill, by taking time off to try other sports. Without variety, "your swimming gets stale and you burn out," she says. "We always did some variety. We would play volleyball, handball, and be playful in the pool. Three times a week, we would run and do additional weight training. Some athletes take off 6 weeks every year, just to get fresh again."

See the correct strokes. Olympic medalist Summer Sanders loves to swim competitively, but she really cherishes her training. "I try to train very hard and simulate a competitive situation every day. I have to concentrate on the end of my training laps because that is where I have problems. When I race, I always get into trouble in the last few meters. I tend to tighten up and not get good distance with my stroke. With my butterfly, I don't get my arms out of the water; I don't extend fully. I try and visualize a full stroke—not a short, quick one, but a full, relaxed one. If I can do this in practice, then it will come naturally in competitive races."

Prepare for race conditions. It's important to prepare both mentally and physically for possible conditions at your events. This is particularly important in mass-start, open-water races such as triathlons, points out Laughlin. "There's the distraction of swimming in open water, plus the distraction of swimming in a knot of people," he says. "You need to go through a rehearsal process, learning how to swim in the open water and concentrate on your technique. I tell triathletes to swim as if there are no other people out there and they're doing a swimming workout."

Tune in to your body. Sanders encourages all swimmers to be aware of their body sensations when they move through the water. "You have to tune in to the movement and the dance of swimming," she says.

Enjoy yourself. Swimmers at any level must approach the sport with a sense of fun and excitement, says Sanders. "You have to love the feel and sensation of the water to learn the basics," she says. "Once you have the understanding that swimming is a creative process, then it becomes easy and

SECRETS OF SUCCESS:
EDDIE REESE

Coach Eddie Reese has been called the world's greatest swimming coach and with a resume at the University of Texas that includes 38 NCAA individual champions, 28 national champion relays, over 150 All-Americans, and 22 Olympians who have won 21 gold medals, few would be inclined to argue.

Reese's ability to technically train his athletes has been a big part of his success. But he also places heavy emphasis on the mental side of training. When we met in Austin, Texas, there was this unusual dynamic that appeared over and over, as he interrupted our conversation to walk poolside and commend his athletes for a strong set of laps. "Nice job, good commitment; I like those times," he bellowed out to his 18- and 19-year-old student athletes.

Reese believes discipline and focus are important; but you must wrap that in the context of mental training. "Each kid must get in the pool each day and see himself win," he says.

Among the techniques Reese preaches, he emphasizes these.

- Work hard, both in the pool and on dry land; you have to visualize your best effort.

- Keep your heart in what you do; love your swimming, and you'll do better.

- Respect your teammates. If you work together and look out for each other, you'll feel stronger and more focused, and you'll ultimately do better.

- Accept with grace the advice and critiques of your coaches and mentors. "I feel that if I can give these kids one little gem each day, something that is relevant to their lives, both in sport and in the real world, I can keep them fresh and focused," Reese says.

lots of fun." Top-ranked triathlete Mike Pigg uses his swim workouts as a time to relax. "Swimming allows me to go into that altered state, that performance zone that is a relaxed, completely focused place," he says.

Schedule time off. Evans reminds all competitors to be sure to listen to their bodies. "If I'm emotionally burned out, then I have to take a few weeks off and get out of the pool," says Evans. "My sophomore year in college I took a little time off, got more into my studies, and became a real person. It was fun to have a social life, but eventually I felt guilty and out of shape, and I knew it was time to return to training."

FOCUS, FOCUS, FOCUS

Competition, of course, is a different arena. In a sport where success depends as much on style as on sheer strength, mental preparation is crucial. Losing your concentration in an 800-meter race or panicking in a triathlon swim when someone accidentally kicks you in the head can drastically affect your finishing time. Here's how to get an edge on the competition.

Learn to relax. The important buzzword for Evans is relaxation. Whatever race she entered, she focused on her goals and her mental preparation, but mostly she stayed very relaxed. "No matter how pumped I was before a race, no matter how important the event, I always reminded myself that I had to be completely relaxed so that my breathing and mental imagery flowed," she says. "If I'm not relaxed, it sets off a negative chain of events."

Find the right tension level. Most swimmers will tell you that the best way to ruin a race is to tighten up. Muscle tension leads directly to shallow breathing, which then increases the anxiety level throughout the body. It's a vicious circle. To break the cycle of tension and increase fluid motion in the water, practice deep, open breathing. Follow that practice session with tight, constrained breathing. Repeating these sequences from tight to relaxed to tight again is a good way to find your rhythm in the water. Evans says it best to her swimming buddies: "You have to take care of your own tension, find the right comfort level, and stay with it."

Choose a narrow focus. "The things that cause anxiety are the things over which you don't believe you have control," says Laughlin. "You can't

SECRETS OF SUCCESS:
JANET EVANS

Have a Life Outside the Water

Retired swim champion and gold-medal Olympian Janet Evans believes strongly in cross-training. She used to run every morning for 30 minutes, lift weights, and do other cross-training. "I had a terrific college roommate, so we tried to have healthy diversions away from swimming," she says. But when it was time to train, she was always ready to go.

When it came time to swim, Evans got serious. She had an enormous work ethic about her training. She also believed in a balanced diet. Before racing, she ate lots of pasta. She insisted on plenty of rest right before a race and, most of all, demanded a positive attitude of herself.

control what other people in the race will do. But the most controllable thing is what you are doing technically. I always told my swimmers to go into a race with one well-focused technical thing to concentrate on. It may be keeping the body balanced or making perfect turns." This helps shut out distractions that you can't control, he says.

Beware of overconfidence. Olympic swimmer Crissy Perham remembers a frustrating loss in Barcelona. "I gave her the race. I couldn't believe that my Chinese competitor was so close to me in the finals at the Barcelona Games. I was, after all, supposed to win. I lost my concentration and my focus, and I wasn't swimming my race. I thought there was no way she could keep up with me; I still wake up in the middle of the night seeing myself finish. I should have had the gold medal. I didn't stay focused but, rather, started visualizing *her* finish." Even in retirement from swimming, she wakes up trying to understand how her imagery shifted from her gold-medal performance to someone else. "I thought about all the wonderful things I would say and do after I won. I not only prepared for the race but I also prepared myself for after the race. I had my speech and the national anthem all worked out in my head. Somehow I just gave it away. I literally looked over into the other lane and gave the race to her. I close my eyes at night and still see that finish."

Follow prerace cues. Perham built in a cue system before every race. She would enter the pool deck, look around and find her parents in the bleachers, throw some "pumpers" (a raised fist in the air), and then make eye contact with her coach. Before racing, she would walk to the podium and touch the first-place spot (where winners stand) and imagine the excitement of receiving her first-place award. Those were her visual and kinesthetic cues.

Find a stress buster. Sanders says that she tries to keep life simple both in training and in competition. "I am a simple, straightforward competitor. I don't go off by myself and do anything fancy before a race. I hang out with my friends and try to be as normal as possible. I laugh a lot; it releases a lot of tension." She was tense and uptight before her first Olympic race in 1992, where she won a bronze, and all the other Olympic races seemed easier after the first one. The pressure was off.

Think positive thoughts. Sanders avoids focusing on negatives; she stays in the present, thinking positive thoughts, saying positive things to herself in the water. During competition, she reminds herself to stay with her game plan. Her biggest temptation is to go on instinct and race someone else at their pace. "Swimming for me is to stay with my game plan, visualizing my full strokes and feeling my pace without getting outside of myself."

Avoid getting psyched out. In Barcelona, 24 hours before the Olympic 200 medley, Sanders was getting nervous. "The rumors were flying about the Chinese women—their strength, their conditioning, their work ethic, and their special herbal enhancements," she says. "It was all very intimidating. For a while I thought these women were amazing—unbeatable! Then I got hold of myself and realized that they were just human beings, other female swimmers just like me. I looked at this one Chinese swimmer, and I said in my own quiet voice, 'She is just a person like me, she is just as nervous, and we are all in it together.' Then I remembered my imagery, my work ethic, the thousands of hours in the pool, the daily double workouts, and my game plan. Once I put the whole thing in perspective and reminded myself about who I was and my strategy for success, then I was ready. No more self-doubt, no more intimidation. I was ready to race."

Bounce back with relaxation and imagery. Sanders did not always have supreme confidence. When she was 14, she struggled with her self-esteem and her swimming. She worked with a psychologist and did some relaxation training as well as imagery practice. "I learned how to relax and do my best," she says. "I also learned not to take the sport so seriously. I would put my goal times up around the house—in the bathroom, in the closet, on the mirrors, and in the hallway. It was a good cue to remind me that I could get there and be successful while relaxed." She also practiced self-talk and positive affirmations before going to the pool. This got her ready and built on her existing confidence. Her biggest mental practice strategy was to visualize her family, friends, and support system. By seeing these people in her mind, it relaxed her and reminded her how far she had come and why it felt so good to be a great swimmer.

Keep your cool. Sanders tries to tell other athletes that competitive swimming is just like a hard practice. She reminds athletes at all levels of competition that racing is not that big a deal. "It is just a swim race. If you just think about it, it is something you have done hundreds of times before; you know how to get the best out of yourself." Just moments before the 400 medley in Barcelona, Sanders was very excited and extremely tense. She reminded herself that she had nothing to lose. She had made it to the Olympic Games, the pinnacle; she could just jump into the pool and have fun. "My first medal was so exciting. I just let it happen. I converted all this anxiety to positive energy. By the 200 medley, I wasn't so excited. I had calmed myself a bit. I converted that tension to toughness and had a heck of a race."

Make plans. In triathlons, the swim is the first of the three events, so Pigg takes full advantage of the time spent in the water to plan the rest of his race. "Swimming offers that additional time to mentally prepare for the other aspects of the competition: the biking and running," he explains. "It also gives me a chance to plan the transitions between the swim, the bike, and the run."

FOR DIVERS ONLY

As a former college gymnast, I can appreciate the intense training and commitment that go into a diver's daily regimen. It is not the rigorous stretching, weight training, and actual diving that is so intense, but rather

(continued on page 176)

SECRETS OF SUCCESS:
NICHOLE HAISLETT-BACHER

Someone who understands the phenomenon of focus is Nicole Haislett (now Haislett-Bacher as of March 2003). She is a real champion and a tough one. She swam in Barcelona in 1992 and at the height of her distinguished career brought home lots of gold. She won triple gold in the 1992 Olympics and one medal in the 200 meters, then won in the 400 free relay and won gold in the medley relay. She finished fourth in the 100 free. She left swimming in 1995 but still stays mentally tough with her aerobic workouts, treadmill runs, weight training, and inline skating.

In preparing for competition, Haislett-Bacher would always structure a relaxation period. "I always did it before my race; I would warm up and just find a quiet spot, put my feet up, and be away from my team," she said, reminiscing about the good ole days. "I would put my headphones on and listen to music and just get mentally prepared."

For focus, Haislett-Bacher would always prepare way ahead of time. "For me, it was easier than other ladies, I think. I had this enormous competitive drive; swimming well and strong was always in my head, but I had to find the right balance, not too much focus, but just enough to keep fine-tuned and ready to go." She explained that for developmental athletes and even college competitors, one has to have a normal life. "You need friends, you need to go out, you have to party with some reasonable limits; have some fun. And don't get overfocused," she told me. But balance is part of being a great competitor. Know your boundaries and your priorities. Haislett-Bacher said that "practice is always the next day, so if you play too hard the night before, you will pay the price, and your coach will make you pay the price, so find the right balance between play and serious commitment to your swimming."

For race time, it was all focus and no play with Haislett-Bacher. Her game face was ready, and she would visualize the game plan each day. "I played the race over and over in my head in order to see myself winning and winning strong. I would visualize a constant routine, see myself accelerating off the wall, my perfect turns, my kick, and my finish. Visualization was very important to me."

Confidence builders for Haislett-Bacher were her starts and turns. "Knowing that I had a good start would build a lot of confidence, and I always reminded myself that the winner is the one with the fewest doubts."

Haislett-Bacher's coach at Florida was a strong influence on her, both as coach and mentor. He helped her take her swimming to the next level. "Mitch Ivey believed in me, believed in my mental preparation, but he was not your standard run-of-the-mill guy. He was unique and didn't go by the book. With him it was tough love for all of us, especially me. He made me think and feel tough; he knew that I needed to step it up, to go to the next level. He had no mercy. He told me I had to stay in top shape, both physically and emotionally. He was a straight shooter, sometimes painfully straight."

Haislett-Bacher emphasizes this coaching relationship with a unique story between coach and athlete. "I was in Canada for a big race. The night before, I fell down some stairs and tore ligaments in my leg; it was serious. I was on crutches. Coach Ivey was upset; he had entered me in an important race; no excuses. He made me swim; he forced me to swim. I threw down the crutches, could barely make my turns or kick, but he made me swim. It definitely redefined mental toughness for me."

Haislett-Bacher's best pointers:

- Learn how to sacrifice.

- Never underestimate hard work.

- Don't be afraid to try new things, but don't get caught up in fad.

- Nutrition is very important; but don't overdo dieting.

- Stay with the basics; stay with fundamentals.

- Be tough mentally, take criticism, and look in the mirror each day and remind yourself that you can handle anything that comes your way.

the mental practice of the event that is so arduous. Divers are, in a sense, gymnasts landing in water. It is the same body movement, the same visual and kinesthetic sense, and the same internal dialogue. Former Olympian Matt Scoggins, diving coach at the University of Texas at Austin, says that many of his divers work out with gymnasts. "In fact, they do quite a bit of work on the trampoline," he says.

When you commit to a rotation in your mind, it needs to be clear and lucid imagery so that the muscle memory will respond with a clear and crisp body movement. If your mind is distracted or cluttered with self-doubt, then the muscle memory and subsequent motions will be cluttered, jerky, and not at all a clean athletic motion. Our minds and bodies are deeply connected. This is true for many sports but certainly punctuated with the sport of diving. If you cannot see or feel yourself in the dive before you do it, it is very unlikely that it will occur with any fluid motion.

As in gymnastics, mental practice and mental imagery control in diving can make or break a performance. You can have the best training in the world, but if you don't practice your mental and visualization strategies, your diving can be mediocre. Competition and the pressures associated with it must be addressed in preparing mentally for great diving. It's one thing to go out to the community pool and show off your double twisting somersaults with your friends. Being put under the spotlight of media, crowd, and judges in an official competition, however, is another issue. The diver who mentally prepares for pressure is the one who can emerge from the water with strong scores.

Divers usually prepare for competitive situations by imaging all the elements that might cause emotional and physiological tension. By visualizing the crowd and the judges, a diver can simulate that tension-anxiety state and perform with some tight leg and upper-body muscles. By practicing in this heightened arousal state, a diver can slowly and progressively learn to relax all the muscles associated with diving technique. This is not a one-shot deal, but a training process that takes place over many years.

Divers also need to overcome fear of the water and build confidence, and for this, Scoggins uses a device called a bubbler. This machine creates a huge mass of bubbles in the water to cushion the diver as he hits the water. "It cushions a bad landing, but more important, it allows our divers to overcome unnecessary fear of a crash," says Scoggins. (When I went down to Austin to see Scoggins and meet his divers, he put the huge bubbler on; it was like a combination tornado and hurricane whipped up into high surf; it looked like a huge white foam milkshake.) When he thinks the divers are ready, and they believe their confidence levels are up and their fear thresholds are down, the bubble machine is turned off.

As with gymnastics training and competition, divers have to be in sync with their coaches. In order to perform a certain element in gymnastics, it was very important for my coach to say to me something like, "Steven, I know what you are feeling up there on the horizontal bar. I also know the sensations of fear, distress, and complete panic that you are going to feel when you release the bar out of your giant swing for a dynamic triple back dismount. I also know the excitement and pleasure you will get from this maneuver. Once you visualize the element and get comfortable in your mind, you will then be able to perform it on the bar." This is the type of dialogue that every gymnast would love to have with his coach. It is the type of communication and trust that you need in order to be able to get to that secure, emotional place—to trust yourself and your imagery that this is all going to work, and work safely.

COACHES—AND PARENTS—PLAY A PART

As the former assistant coach at the University of Arizona in Tucson, Crissy Perham spent time with her athletes discussing issues of fear: fear of winning, fear of losing, and fear of failure as an elite athlete. Under the mentorship of swimming coach Frank Bush, Perham grew to love swimming and the competitive spirit that goes with the territory. Her struggle was with training and the long hours. She loved to compete and looked forward to a tough race, but she had to deal with the discipline of long workouts. As a coach, she was aware that there had to be a balance of both.

"I think that my natural inclination was to go out there and kick some butt in a race," she says. "I enjoyed the whole process. During the warmups and the introductions and in the waiting room before we were called, I used to love the excitement and the anticipation. Some athletes get hyper, superaroused, and completely freaked out before competition. That was not my problem. I used to clown around, step on people's thongs, play music, and boogie in the locker room. I enjoyed getting juiced up before the big competitions. What I learned as a coach was that other athletes have different styles of coping and dealing with the stress of competition. I think that it is very important to honor and respect those individual differences."

Perham notes that confidence is a big issue with swimmers. Some need to have constant support and reinforcement. She believes that competitors derive their training and competition styles from their childhoods and their family support systems. "My parents never let me quit swimming, and yet they never forced me to compete or imposed their will about being serious with the sport. They were just there in the background as supportive parents without the threat of coercion. It makes a difference in what a child brings to his sport based on his parental influence."

Her parents were important role models, and Perham attributes her success to the fact that they encouraged her to have fun and not take swimming too seriously. She says that when pushy parents cause problems, their kids may succeed in sports, but they lack any real enjoyment or fulfillment in their accomplishments.

WORKSHEET: MENTAL TRAINING
FOR SWIMMING AND DIVING

Whether you compete in swim meets, triathlons, or diving competitions—or just swim recreationally—you can benefit from mental training. Review these techniques before your workouts or competitions. You'll want to customize these to meet your own goals and needs and take note of what images or techniques work best for you.

Use affirmations and self-talk. Practice these during training as well as racing. Tell yourself during a tough race or workout, "I can do this." Don't allow negative thoughts such as "Those other swimmers look awfully strong" or "I don't think I can make up the time I need." If you have a bad start, a poor turn, or a less-than-perfect dive, tell yourself, "Stay calm; put it behind you." Choose a cue word or phrase such as "You can do it" to use in tough spots during the competition.

Breathe right. Practice full breathing regularly (see Chapter 4 for specific practice steps). Before your race, you may want to listen to a specific piece of music to practice relaxed, comfortable breathing. You might want to pair an image, such as making a graceful flip-turn or finishing a race well, with your breathing routine.

Meditate. Meditation during a race or training will help you shut out the outside world and concentrate on your own race. You might choose a mantra such as "Stay calm; stay steady" to repeat before and during the race to help you concentrate and stay relaxed.

Relax. After hard workouts, practice progressive relaxation to relax your muscles. Establish your own relaxation routine with an audiotape. Practice a mini relaxation session, perhaps taking deep breaths or counting backward from 10 to calm yourself or relax overly tense muscles. Practice relaxing during workouts so you can call up the relaxation response between events, if needed.

Practice imagery and visualization. To begin guided imagery, identify how you view images by filling out the questionnaire on page 56. For imagery practice, watch film clips of competitions or instructional tapes. You'll find a guided imagery program on page 240.

Consider your opponents. Some athletes visualize opponents. Some see all the competition and feel very queasy. Evans overcame that by shifting the scenery and imaging all her opponents as enemies so she could get on with her game plan. This worked; she became a great swimmer and a very tough competitor.

Visualize technique. Technique is crucial in swimming. A hand placed in the water incorrectly or a botched flip-turn could cost you the race. In your mind, watch yourself during a competition, slow down your visualization, and correct any mistakes you see. Your best tools are videotapes of yourself swimming so you can easily identify and correct errors in your style via mental and physical practice.

Build a victory image. Imagine yourself winning your event; feel the sensation of a strong finish and hear the sounds. If you're a triathlete, see yourself coming out of the water strong and sprinting up the beach. If you're a competitive swimmer or diver, see yourself finishing well and seeing the finish clock or final scoring and perhaps pumping your fist in the air in a victory salute.

Use visual motor behavior rehearsal (VMBR). Visualize yourself in a competition; focus on enhancing your technique and analyzing and mentally correcting errors. If your flip-turns are poor, practice them in your mind until you do them smoothly and without error. While training, practice the corrected behavior. Before races, imagine all the details of the race

---

SECRETS OF SUCCESS: SUMMER SANDERS

Have Fun—And Remember Your Successes

Olympic medalist Summer Sanders has retired from swimming, but she still talks to young competitors about her mental training strategies. She tells kids to have fun, enjoy the sport, and work hard at it. She reminds athletes to go to practice and to practice perfectly. "Don't just go through the motions; focus and concentrate on what you're doing. Practice as if it were the biggest race of your life. Don't just hang out in the pool. Put in good, solid workouts."

Sanders has a delightful way of reminding people that competitive swimming should be fun: You just go out there, shut out the world, and enjoy your race, she says. When she talks to high school students about swimming, she reminds them of the basics. "First and foremost, swim for yourself. Don't do it for Mom or Dad," she says. "Next, remember to stay with your game plan; don't get sucked into someone else's race strategy. Remember next that you are all great competitors at any level, and you are all human beings and have vulnerabilities. Finally, recall your imagery from training, your work ethic, and your hard and fast finishes; have that supreme confidence when you train and bring it with you when you race."

---

and how you will meet challenges that might arise, such as feeling pain, having cramps, or feeling inadequate or unprepared. Practice switching back and forth between a relaxed phase and a ready-to-win state of mind (see page 65 for specific steps).

Have a precompetition routine. Anticipate, prepare for, and minimize as many distractions as possible. At the race site, check out the surroundings, the crowd, the weather (if your race or meet is outside), and the noise. Look around to see who your competitors are. Thirty minutes before race time, move into your PTEZ, or perfect timing and energy zone. Practice relaxed breathing. Visualize yourself swimming during the competition, dealing with adversity such as pain and fatigue, and finishing strongly. Tell yourself that you will do well in this race. Do any prerace rituals that make you more comfortable.

Unlike other swimmers who need quiet and private time before competition, Perham gets goofy and loves to begin her competitive ritual by

<hr />

SECRETS OF SUCCESS:
JUSTIN DUMAIS

Keep It in the Family

Diving is not just a sport or passion for Justin Dumais, it is a familial right of passage. "My brother Troy competed with me in college (at the University of Texas, Austin), my brother Brice competes at Southern Methodist, my sister Leanne will be diving for Northwestern in the fall of 2003, and the youngest one, Dwight, is diving in high school." Coming from parents who played tennis and softball and instilled a strong work ethic in all five kids, the Dumais family has some strong DNA when it comes to sports. Especially water sports.

"My parents are very focused, very conservative and religious, so yes, they gave us strong values around discipline and competition," says Dumais, the recipient of 13 national championships, five international titles, and many more honors including third at the 2003 Pan Am Games.

Dumais's command of the mental aspects of diving is a big part of his competitive advantage. He claims to have "stupid smarts"—the ability to turn off his brain and let doubt disappear. "I can win it if I let my mind go," he says.

Here's his recipe for diving success.

- Get plenty of rest. Confidence fails when your body is fatigued.

- Run through your tape in your head.

- Focus on one technique.

- Don't visualize during competition, only during training.

- Repeat a mantra. Dumais's is "I'm the best."

stepping on everyone's thongs on the pool deck. Other rituals may include playing a song in your head, meditating, or talking to other athletes. Some athletes like to distract themselves from the setting, while others stay very present and focused. Either way, use your own personal ritual to get the most out of your precompetition strategy.

CHAPTER 18

Tennis: Keep Your Cool on the Court

In the tennis world, Nick Bollettieri is a legend. Need proof? Here's a small list of athletes he's worked with: Andre Agassi, Aaron Krickstein, Jim Courier, Kathleen Horvath, Carling Bassett, Pete Sampras, Monica Seles, Mary Pierce, Martina Hingis, Tommy Haas, Mark Philipoussis, Venus and Serena Williams, Anna Kournikova, and Boris Becker.

Kind of leaves you breathless. But talk with Bollettieri and he'll tell you that it isn't the skills these athletes possess that make them standouts. It's their passion—their mental focus on the game.

"I have worked with some of the greatest athletes in the world over 30 years, but none of that matters if they don't have the love, the positive attitude, and the passion to play and care for the game," he says. "Winning at that level is all about attitude, passion, and respect for the game."

Sport psychologist Jim Loehr, PhD, founding director of sport sciences for the United States Tennis Association and cofounder of LGE Sport Science Training Center in Orlando, Florida, gives credence to Bollettieri's beliefs. Frame of mind is directly linked with performance, he says.

"Mental and emotional mistakes we make in one motor movement translate into physiological problems across the board," he says. "It is important to never separate the mind from the body in things we do."

To prove this point, we need look no further than Bollettieri's student and perhaps the best tennis player ever, Pete Sampras.

As a young rising tennis star, top-seeded tennis champion Sampras struggled with maintaining his concentration and controlling his frustration and anger on the court. "I would lose my composure and sometimes completely blow it on the court," he told me several years ago. "My dad, who was coaching me then, was very strict and basically told me that my tennis career was history if I didn't pull myself together. I also learned early on that having a tantrum on the court was very embarrassing and looks pretty bad. The other part of the emotional control equation was that when I had a flare-up, it was very hard to rebound and get back in the game. My temper got in the way of being in a focused tennis mind; it became very destructive."

SECRETS OF A TOP PLAYER

Sampras, who was the number one–ranked tennis player in the world in 1994, learned his lessons well. Although he just stepped down and retired in September 2003, he is one of those rare athletes who appears to stay in total control on the court, regardless of the situation. He reminds young players that they must understand the dynamics of their emotions, especially anger, before they move to the next level of competitive play. Here are some ways that he maintains his concentration during play.

Keep things uncomplicated. "I try and keep my strategy simple," Sampras says. "I stay very intense during a match and completely focused. I never think about an opponent until the moment we play, and then my focus is on where to serve and how to hit crosscourt and down the line. I try not to complicate my life by spending too much time analyzing a player in advance."

Concentrate. Tennis is all about concentration and staying focused in the moment, says Sampras. "My most difficult match is when I am winning a series of points easily—too easily—and I lose my concentration. I forget what I'm doing momentarily with a brain fade, and then I lose my edge. I pay for it with the next several points."

Channel your emotions. The key to good tennis is to stay relaxed, yet focused, and to maintain a good balance between the highs and lows, according to Sampras. "I get very upset when I miss a point that is important, but I keep that upset within me," he says. "When I get a bad call by a line judge, my upset goes ballistic, but again, I keep that well contained. In order to play well, you have to learn to channel the emotions, both the highs and the very lows."

Let yourself move on. Sampras plays a little head game with himself to get over his mishaps. He tells himself after a missed shot, "I need to move on to the next point; I should not be in this position." After that mantra, he

MENTAL MASTERS

Nick Bollettieri is one of the leading figures in the sport of tennis, as coach, mentor, promoter, and author. He is founder of the Bollettieri IMG Training Center in Bradenton, Florida, and coauthor with Julie Anthony, PhD, of *Winning Combination: A Parents' Guide to Tennis.*

David Higdon, a former nationally ranked college tennis player, is a sports-writer for several US magazines. He is now vice president of corporate communications for the Association of Tennis Professionals (ATP).

Jim Loehr, PhD, is a sport psychologist, ranked senior player, and the founding director of sport sciences for the United States Tennis Associ-ation. He is cofounder of LGE Sport Science Training Center in Orlando, Florida, and has written 11 books on the subject of sport psychology.

Chad Bohling is the mental rehearsal and training skill builder behind the brilliance of Nick Bollettieri. He runs the "mental conditioning depart-ment" of the Bollettieri Academy in Bradenton, Florida. As a graduate of Wichita State University in Wichita, Kansas, a varsity tennis player, and then on to San Diego State University in San Diego for a masters degree, Bohling knows a bit or two about mental training and peak performance.

Pete Sampras turned pro at age 16. He was the 1990 US Open Cham-pion at 19 and was the number one–ranked tennis player in the world in 1994. He retired from tennis on the first night of the 2003 US Open in New York City during a very emotional ceremony carried live around the globe. He has 65 career single titles and 14 grand slam wins.

never thinks about the last point. It is gone, history, time to refocus on the present.

Find the right coach. Pete Fisher, MD, a Los Angeles pediatrician, coached Sampras from age 8 to 16. Dr. Fisher became a mentor and was instrumental in Sampras's career. "Often parents are well-meaning, but they can put too much pressure on a kid," Sampras told me. "For me, it was important to have a family friend in Dr. Fisher, who could help me with the emotional/psychological aspect of tennis and yet give me pointers to improve my game. I think my dad was incredibly supportive, but it was important for an outsider to step in and guide me."

SECRETS OF SUCCESS: JIM LOEHR

Tips from a Top Tennis Consultant

Sport psychologist Jim Loehr, PhD, founding director of sport sciences for the United States Tennis Association, cofounder of LGE Sport Science Training Center in Orlando, Florida, and consultant to Gabriela Sabatini and other stars, offers this prescription for great tennis.

• Learn to isolate factors such as physiological arousal or the ideal performance state.

• Learn to balance your energy and state of arousal. You don't want to be too aroused, or you'll lose control. Likewise, you don't want to be underaroused, where you are too laid back and don't get up for the match. Pretend that you are an actor or actress and learn to control arousal states. Actors typically get deep into their emotional states to prepare for the shooting of a movie, and tennis is very similar to this process.

• Be prepared to look carefully at the sequence between your tennis points. Sport scientists say that this is the critical moment where matches are won or lost. When the point is over, tennis experts look at how athletes hold their heads, how they walk, their demeanor, and how

SCIENCE AT WORK

Dr. Loehr knows about the relationship of muscle tension to the smooth flow and rhythm necessary in competitive tennis. His major goal since the 1970s has been to educate people about the relationship of the mind to the body in the context of sport and to demystify mental training strategies. Dr. Loehr says that athletes and coaches often are too hung up on the supposed stigma to have a sport psychologist or consultant assist their game.

"We need to reeducate the coaching community that sport is really about the integration of sport science with the actual playing of the game," Dr.

they move to the next sequence of activity. If you hold the racket too tightly or your jaw is clenched and you are ruminating about the last point that you messed up, then your muscles and emotional memory will contaminate the next series of points.

Dr. Loehr and other tennis experts try to get athletes to see this critical period on videotape. "I want my young, old, amateur, and pro tennis players to see this sequence so that they can experience firsthand their emotions during this in-between-point period," he explains. "If we can get them to rid themselves of those 3½ seconds of negativity, hold their heads high, achieve new self-confidence, and prepare for the next point with a clean physiological and emotional slate, then we have done good work in our training.

"Often, when athletes can learn to relax between points, they will drop 16 to 20 points in their heart rates during this recovery period," says Dr. Loehr. That translates into a 20 percent increase in their physical and emotional preparation states for the next point. And if you keep training with the mind-body connection between each point, you raise an enormous level of awareness among competitors about the entire pace of a 3-hour match."

Loehr says. "What I have tried to do over many years is take the best players in the tennis world and study them intensively. I study their behavior from the moment they tie their sneakers and warm up until they finish their training. I analyze their breathing, their body language, how they hold their rackets, and what expressions they have on their faces at different stages of play. We are very scientific about our training strategies in tennis."

One of the key areas for Dr. Loehr is understanding stress in young athletes. He looks immediately for stress points and how individuals manage their stress. "If we take the top 20 seeds in the world and videotape them and analyze their attitudes and physical mechanisms toward stress management, we can learn a whole lot," he says. "What you will see in the top 20 players will be vastly different from what you'll observe in the 21st through 50th international rankings."

Dr. Loehr and his colleagues use high-speed cinematography to evaluate every motion, every tic, and every idiosyncrasy within a player. They study the biomechanics of the individual and then look critically at the strokes to see if they fit the physiology of the athlete. Their training institute uses electrocardiograms (EKGs) and wireless heart monitors to understand what happens internally when the player is resting between points. They also look at vital signs when the athlete is engaged in competitive battle. Dr. Loehr says that if the heart rate stays high between points (during the resting and recovery zone), then the player is overstressed and headed for early burnout in the match. "The optimal condition between points is a stress/recovery balance, such that the heart rate is typically falling between points, the player is relaxed biomechanically, and the breathing returns to normalcy," he says. "Otherwise, if the EKG is up, the body will be tense, and that translates into tight muscle-reflex action and some bad tennis."

Chad Bohling, who runs the "mental conditioning department" of the Bollettieri Academy in Bradenton, Florida, agrees with this type of psychological/physiological profiling. "It works with everyone, from high school to collegiate to Olympian to pro athlete," he says. "Everyone has a technique, a style. We try not to mess with that, just tweak it a bit, but on the mental conditioning side, there is lots of work that can be done. We have a three-prong approach in our tennis training: technique, physical performance, and mental training."

These methods have worked so well for Bollettieri players that they now use them to train soccer players and basketball and baseball stars. Just recently, the NFL's Jacksonville Jaguars tapped them to train its players.

THE SAGA OF SABATINI

Former professional tennis star Gabriela Sabatini, who was consistently ranked in the top five female professional players in the world, was one of Dr. Loehr's shining stars. She sought the professional services of Dr. Loehr and his staff after struggling for many years to achieve the pinnacle of success. In a *World Tennis* magazine article, Dr. Loehr describes his very focused and structured intervention with Sabatini, calling her evolution from an elite tennis star to the best in the world "the most engaging and dramatic story" with which he had ever been associated.

Dr. Loehr believed it was crucial to have the entire Sabatini family present, plus her coach and trainer, to become part of the training process so that Sabatini would have as much emotional support as possible. Although Sabatini is bilingual, her family was encouraged to debrief all training sessions in Spanish so that all family members could discuss her feelings and emotions openly and carefully. Off the court, Dr. Loehr encouraged her to write down her goals clearly and succinctly so that she could reflect on them and add to them when necessary.

One of Sabatini's fears was that she would retire from tennis without ever reaching her ultimate goal: a major international title. Knowing that emotions are so tied to one's tennis game and court demeanor, Dr. Loehr created a videotape of footage from Sabatini's best matches and put them to her favorite music. With her own personalized music video, Sabatini was instructed to watch her best forehands, backhands, volleys, serve-and-volleys, and returns of serve as often as possible.

Knowing that external stimuli often enhance the quality of our internal imagery machines, Dr. Loehr wanted to strengthen Sabatini's sense of internal imagery and boost her self-confidence. He also wanted her to let go emotionally on the court, releasing some of the anger, frustration, joy, and elation that she was used to holding onto. The music video was a vehicle to bring freshness to her game and her passion and identity as a player and simultaneously strengthen her visual and auditory senses. Dr. Loehr also became sensitized to another important element in the training equation, her family.

SECRETS OF SUCCESS:
PETE SAMPRAS

Four Steps to Great Tennis

Tennis great Pete Sampras says there are four gifts that he would bestow on any young player.

- Know thyself. Know that you have the complete power to win, or you can choose to lose.

- Take control of a competitive situation. Know your strengths and your weaknesses on the court.

- Be realistic about your goals; don't expect too much too soon.

- Find a coach who works best for you. Don't be afraid to change coaches if the fit is not a good one.

Sabatini needed to know that her parents and her brother (who came often to training sessions) would be there for her, win or lose. Dr. Loehr encouraged the family to reach out emotionally to Sabatini as she scripted her goals and renewed her confidence in her quest for a championship. Conversely, he encouraged Sabatini to take greater risks with her coach, trainer, and family members. Dr. Loehr encouraged unconditional love, support, and acceptance for everyone involved. He wanted Sabatini to know that she could be tough and aggressive on the court and simultaneously loved for who she is, no matter what the outcome of her matches.

In 1990, Sabatini had a major breakthrough at the US Open: She beat Leila Meshki in the quarters, Mary Jo Fernandez in the semifinals, and then Steffi Graf for the title. Her mental training had paid off.

MANAGING ANGER AND ANXIETY

One of the other major influences on the game of tennis is anger and how it is managed. Many amateur and professional athletes carry anger around with them and are able to use it to their advantage. In football, for instance, a lineman may use the power of his rage to hit two blockers and then sack the quarterback. This may be great on the gridiron, but in tennis it could create many problems. Tennis is a delicate fine-motor sport, and all motions are influenced by the athlete's emotional states. Anger may certainly undermine this delicate motor process. Anxiety can undermine the process as well, especially if there is no outlet for it. Some athletes take anxiety and convert it into rage. In some sports, this is socially acceptable and appropriate, but in tennis, it isn't. Here's how some top athletes deal with anxiety.

Redirect your stress. Some athletes get so anxious before competition that they have no idea what to do with their stress. Some turn inward and get physically sick, and others turn outward and release it into the external world. Tennis great Jimmy Connors had much anxiety before matches and over time learned to release it in a healthy, socially acceptable way. In his early days, he had screaming outbursts at the officials; but later in his career, he turned the anxiety into some very creative antics on the court. He would usually convert anger and anxiety into some odd face or body motion and get lots of positive energy and enjoyment out of it. John McEnroe, however, struggled with the conversion process and never learned how to convert all this anxiety and tension into something pleasurable. Over many years, he did get some effective use out of his anger as he deflected it into the crowd. He may have won points and matches utilizing this tactic, but he didn't win over many friends or fans. And he got his share of monetary fines for some of his behavior on the court.

Keep your rhythm. The more important issue at stake here is what happens when you lose control (either by choice or inadvertently) and your game starts to deteriorate. The game of tennis is so interconnected to the mind and body that it is nearly impossible to not affect the physiology when you have a bad emotional moment, says tennis pro Len Spencer. "Tennis is all about a psychological rhythm, which then sets off a muscle and correct tension flow," he explains. "If you are upset about your serve, invariably that emotion will translate into poor muscle control and a ball that is out of bounds. If you hit two poor serve-and-volleys in a row, that will translate into a negative muscle memory and increased body tightness."

Change the chemistry. Most experts suggest that when the emotions of anger and rage start to emerge in a young athlete, the goal should be

SECRETS OF SUCCESS:
CHAD BOHLING

Videotaping is one of the best mental training techniques a tennis player can use, according to Chad Bohling, who routinely films students of the Bollettieri IMG Training Academy. "We need to have you see yourself on tape, then learn from that," he says. "One of the more poignant examples of using video for improvement in the mental imagery game is for rehab and with athletes coming off injuries. Athletes coming off injuries and surgery are frustrated, their self-esteem is low, and they need to *see* progress."

For example, when Tommy Haas tore his rotator cuff and needed surgery in 2002, Bohling used video to help him see the small improvements in his rehab. This let Haas see that he was improving over time, even if he couldn't tell day to day.

"He knows that he is making strides toward recovery, which builds in more self-confidence and a quicker healing process," Bohling said at the time. "It's all part of the emotional/physical/psychological paradigm, and we know it works."

to reduce the chemistry of this emotion and change the perception of what is happening. We know that with every emotion (both positive and negative) there is a chemical reaction that responds physiologically. For example, in a fine-motor sport like tennis, if you get the wrong chemicals cooking throughout your bloodstream, you could find yourself in trouble. The trick is to change the scenery, the understanding of the situation, and the perception of losing and winning and realize that the game is only a game. The arousal mechanism in tennis is so delicate that you have to go into the game understanding your arousal state. If you are playing in a friendly weekend doubles tournament with your spouse and you had a bad argument the night before, your emotions will affect your tennis. Unless you are skilled enough to channel the energy of rage, resentment, and upset into a booming serve-and-volley, you are in for a difficult afternoon.

MORE ON THE ANGER SYNDROME

Sport science professionals and coaches agree that the greatest attribute in a rising tennis star is being able to manage anger and channel frustration and disappointment into a positive state of mental preparation. Easier said than done. Dr. Loehr points out that he has lost some great players over the years to the anger syndrome.

"I have worked with the most talented athletes in the world, and some have gone on to win the US Open, Wimbledon, the Australian, the French, and the Grand Slam," he says. But "some athletes are not willing to look at this issue and address its roots, causes, and manifestations. It takes time and energy to deal with emotional issues, and some kids just don't want to take the time to do that. The real key with anger management is to work with the coach, the parents, and the athletes simultaneously. Everyone has to be in the loop—no secrets, no hidden agendas—complete disclosure with everyone present. I try and get everyone in the room together to confront these issues, and then we work together to construct positive solutions."

Find your focus. "Tennis is about 90 percent mental," says former nationally ranked college tennis player David Higdon, sports writer for several US magazines and now a senior vice president for the Association of Tennis Professionals (ATP). "Once you throw your racket on the court or 'lose it' in some other way, it's very hard to regain that control. Composure is so fundamental in this game." Higdon has studied the best and brightest in the tennis world and knows their faults, idiosyncrasies, and rituals. "Tennis is such a focused game," he says. "You look at someone like McEnroe. He is the best study in total concentration. The guy could throw his racket, cuss out the officials, and have a complete tennis tantrum, and within seconds be 110 percent back in focus and in the game. But that's rare. To return to a rhythm and a focused composure in tennis is difficult after a major distraction." Higdon suggests that McEnroe might be the most outstanding player of his time in this regard. "Not that I would encourage a young student athlete to get out of control, but I do admire his complete mental focus and shift from one extreme to the other at a moment's notice."

Turn to outside influences. There are other influences on the anger-rage dilemma, says Higdon. "When my father or any other family member came to watch me play in college, I had more control; I had to have the control," he explains. "I didn't want to embarrass myself and shame the family name. I knew that there would be consequences for getting out of control, so I would always monitor my on-court behavior when my folks were there. But, of course, as soon as my parents were gone, it was a different story. The same was true with my coach. When he was around, I played better, with more control and with my head in the game. When he wasn't watching, I felt alone out there—isolated, not in control, and resentful. I remember losing a big finals in college when my coach went to another court to watch another guy play. I felt abandoned, alone, and resentful that he wasn't there for me."

Fit the strategy to the athlete. What works for one may not be the best mental training strategy or the most appropriate for another athlete. In the game of tennis, proper decorum is one issue, but finesse is another key factor. Psychologists have tried to analyze McEnroe's strategies, including his blind rages, for many years. One noted expert has suggested that McEnroe used the energy of a tantrum or rage to get himself back in the game after a brief slump or a bad run of serves. By getting himself upset, he was able to pump the adrenaline, tap into his quick energy source flowing from anger, and then channel it. Another theorist has suggested that McEnroe's strategies were more devious and in fact quite complex as a competitive strategy. Some say that he used blind rage as a distraction to the crowd and the television audience and ultimately created a circus atmosphere that would adversely affect his opponent. The embarrassment and humiliation that he brought on himself were deflected to others so that the massive confusion on the court got everyone out of sync. Be aware, though, that while top-ranked players may have these psychological factors down to a science, an amateur who attempts similar antics is more apt to end up simply looking foolish.

THE RIGHT BLEND OF CIVILITY AND AGGRESSION

Another product of the LGE Sport Science Training Center was tennis professional Shuzo Matsuoka, the first Japanese player ever to be ranked on the men's professional circuit. According to Dr. Loehr, Matsuoka was struggling with his game, was not well integrated with his biomechanics, and lacked self-confidence when he came to the United States to train. "We put his entire demeanor on videotape: his walk, his body language, his strokes,

SECRETS OF SUCCESS:
ODED TEIG

Spending 3 years as the number one player at one of the nation's top tennis programs taught Oded Teig a few things about handling anger and frustration and putting the needs of his team before his own feelings.

His contribution to the team was more than just wins. He provided a stability and an anchor to the emotional side of his play and that of his players. "I had a lot of times when I was angry and frustrated on the court," he told me recently. "In most cases, I just tried to hold my thoughts for a second and think about positive things and how great it would be to change the outcome of the match when I was up and down," he said. "I also tried to remember how much fun I am having when I am playing good and relaxed, without thinking about the score. I sometimes understand that I can't play my best tennis on any given day. It just has to flow, and you can't push the envelope with tennis."

His record bears out the good this did him: He won 13 out of 15 in Pac-10 matches and won a total of 69 singles matches for a new Oregon collegiate school record. Teig was ranked as high as 15th in doubles and as high as 73rd in singles in the Intercollegiate Tennis Association (ITA) rankings.

Making all this easier was Teig's coach at Oregon, Chris Russell.

"Coach Russell always tried to support me and cheer me on during matches," he says. "When I was down in a match, he always told me how much confidence he has in me and my game and that I can turn things around if I will take one point at a time. He always reminded me that he knows that I am the man and that I can carry the team—those comments always gave me enormous confidence. He also understood that I like to be by myself and be my own person during matches, and he respected that."

But the best mental tip Teig can give for developing athletes and young players is this: Love the game with all your heart. "Acknowledge how fortunate you are to play the game and have access to courts and coaches and good teachers," he says. "Work hard even when it's not so comfortable and always learn and want to improve your game."

his serve, and his critical between-point behavior," says Dr. Loehr. "It was a mess. Basically, Matsuoka was too polite. He was a product of his wonderful culture—very gracious." This exceedingly polite behavior adversely affected Matsuoka's game, and he needed to learn to adopt certain on-court attributes to let him reach his goal of being among the top 50 players in the world.

After 7 months of rigorous training, Matsuoka had a tremendous breakthrough. Dr. Loehr and company isolated the various stages of his play and had him mentally rehearse the corrections of those stages. They examined his fear of other players as well as his balance, coordination, heart rate, and ability to change his demeanor on the court. They led him to examine his own emotions and allowed him to see that his polite and courteous behavior set off chemical reactions that did not permit a powerful down-the-line or crosscourt shot. "We let him transform his body language, posture, and emotions so that this energy could be channeled into a new confidence on the court," says Dr. Loehr. It was a stunning success—Matsuoka's rankings improved dramatically.

Whether it is anger management or just the implementation of mental practice training, tennis experts all agree that parents must be a key factor in the development of young tennis athletes. There has to be support from all components of the coach, consultant, and parent team, with much love and understanding from the parents first. The healthiest players come from families that initially pushed their kids but, as they progressed, allowed them to examine their strengths in collaboration with a coach. Like the motor movements of tennis, the training and mental practice side is also a delicate balance.

WORKSHEET: MENTAL TRAINING FOR TENNIS

Review the following mental training techniques before your next tennis game or practice session. You'll want to customize these tools to meet your own goals and needs and take note of what images or techniques work best for you.

Use affirmations and self-talk. Practice these during training as well as during your game. Tell yourself during a tough match or practice, "I can do this." Don't allow negative thoughts such as "That other player looks stronger than me" or "I don't think I can make up the points I need." If you have a poor serve or miss a return, stay calm and move on. Choose a cue word or phrase such as "You can do it" to use in tough spots during the competition.

Breathe right. Practice full breathing regularly (see Chapter 4 for specific practice steps). Before your game, you may want to listen to a specific piece of music to practice relaxed, comfortable breathing. You might want to pair an image, such as making a spectacular and graceful return, with your breathing routine.

Meditate. Meditation during a workout or competition will help you shut out the outside world and concentrate on your own match. You might choose a mantra such as Sampras's "Move on to the next point; I should not be in this position" to help you concentrate and stay relaxed.

Relax. After hard workouts, practice progressive relaxation to relax your muscles. Establish your own relaxation routine with an audiotape. Practice relaxing during workouts so you can call up the relaxation response before and after play and so you don't tense up before or between games. You may also want to develop a mini relaxation routine, perhaps taking a few deep breaths or counting backward from 10, to calm yourself as needed during play. You need to be revved up to a certain extent to compete, but over-arousal or excessive tension can lead to poor play. Only you—and your coach, if you have one—can determine what the optimal tension level is for you.

Practice imagery and visualization. To begin guided imagery, identify how you view images by filling out the questionnaire on page 56. For imagery practice, watch film clips of major events such as Wimbledon or instructional tennis videotapes. You'll find a guided imagery program on page 240.

Consider your opponent. Loehr tells all his students, including Sabatini, Sampras, and Jennifer Capriati, that they must know something about the person across the net. In fact, it is most useful to pick out the strongest shot or aspect of their game. Know that information about your opponent and stash it away on your internal hard drive.

Visualize technique. In your mind, watch yourself playing and slow down your visualization and correct any mistakes you see. (Videotape is a great tool here.) Watch yourself serving and returning; study your footwork and the position of your arms and body. Identify the areas that need correcting and begin to work on them, both in your mind and on the practice court.

Build a victory image. The great matches of all time have left us with some enduring imprints: Connors falling to his knees after a win at Wimbledon; Martina Navratilova throwing kisses to her fans at the US Open; Sampras embracing his opponent as he wins at the Australian; Andre Agassi ripping off his sweaty shirt and tossing it into the crowd at the French Open. You can get inspiration from these images, but form your own victory image, with your own victory salute, and enjoy the feeling that comes with it.

Use visual motor behavior rehearsal (VMBR). Visualize yourself in a match; focus on enhancing your technique and analyzing and mentally correcting errors. If you lose your temper, practice watching yourself remain calm. If you routinely muff a certain type of return, practice a smooth, sure return. While training, practice the corrected behavior. Before matches, imagine all the details of the competition and how you will meet challenges that might arise. Practice switching back and forth between a relaxed phase and a ready-to-win state of mind (see page 65 for specific steps).

Have a pregame routine. Anticipate, prepare for, and minimize as many distractions as possible. At the competition site, check out the surroundings, the crowd, the weather, and the noise. Size up your opponent and think about what you know about your opponent's playing style, strengths, and weaknesses. Thirty minutes before game time, move into your PTEZ, or perfect timing and energy zone. Practice relaxed breathing. Visualize yourself serving cleanly, making sharp returns, and overcoming adversity. Tell yourself that you will do well in this competition. Do any pre-event rituals that make you more comfortable. These may include listening to music, doing a relaxation routine, watching a video, tying your shoelaces over and over again, or even hugging a favorite teddy bear. Sabatini's ritual is to relax and play lots of videotape and music (like a personal music video session) before she gets on the court.

CHAPTER 19

Volleyball: Correct the Flaws in Your Game

In volleyball, you have a brief window of time to read defense, anticipate play, communicate with your teammates—and get to the ball. In both recreational and competitive volleyball, the secret of good play is mental training. While it's ideal to have someone videotape your game so you can analyze your play and improve every step of the way, you can improve as a volleyball player even without that advantage.

PREPARE FOR THE GAME

Olympic bronze medalist Yoko Zetterlund plays volleyball with great intensity. An American who grew up in Japan, for most of her life she knew only one sport. The Japanese sports system is rigorous, and when you are selected to play a sport, you play that sport exclusively. "I really love this game, and I cherish practice, training, and the discipline associated with volleyball," she says. "I think about touching the ball every day, and I enjoy the team camaraderie and the feeling of working cohesively. I could not play this game so intensively if I didn't love it."

Zetterlund does mental practice—a lot of mental practice. She and her teammates scope out opponents to better understand the dynamics of team interaction. They look for mistakes, flaws, and lack of flow in their own game as they review slow-motion tape. They critique their ball handling and setups and know where there are deficiencies in the game. "We also meet one-on-one with our coaches to understand the positioning of the setters, hitters, and spikers," she explains. "We examine our roles on the court, the placement of our feet, and our body motion. We use the videotape to initiate the visual and kinesthetic feedback and then support that with verbal feedback from our coaching staff." Here's how Zetterlund, other elite players, and a top coach mentally prepare for games.

Increase body awareness. Former Olympian and assistant coach of the US Men's Olympic Volleyball Team Rudy Suwara was a high school gymnast but shifted to volleyball when he started to grow. "I think that the body control and general kinesthetic awareness from gymnastics helped me with my volleyball skills," he says. "I encourage all of our Olympians to work out with a trampoline to fine-tune that body awareness." If you don't have access to a trampoline, you can do workouts on a minitrampoline that will help. Other body awareness–building activities include dance and tai chi.

Visualize position. Top US volleyball player Lori Endicott, member of the 1996 Olympic Volleyball Team and a former top-ranked player at the University of Nebraska in Lincoln, is meticulous about physical as well as mental preparation for all her matches. "I review the same way for each competition," she says. "I go over the game plan that the coaches have put together. I check the scouting report. Our whole team watches videos, and we observe the six rotations. We look at the possibilities of each rotation, where all six athletes could and should be on the court."

Anticipate the action. Suwara and other great players and coaches say the best athletes are the ones who anticipate the unexpected. They are the ones who take time to review the tapes and then practice on their own. "I have some players who come in and watch where their hands are on the net," says Suwara. "They watch the action of the spikers and their approach and observe facial expressions in anticipation of the ball rotation. The defensive decisions have to be made early on. We run the film at 32 frames per second, so we break it down to moment-to-moment energy and anticipate split-second response time."

Know your opponents. Endicott is definitely a student of the game. "Each team has tendencies for each rotation; the offense they run can be different on each rotation," she says. "Certain players have different styles of setting and hitting from various distances along the net." Endicott checks the scouting report before an international competition to see where opponents hit from. She also knows who the good passers are and who is best to serve to. She and teammates break down the action with slow motion and analyze the flow of the game. They also focus on specific players, how they hit and who receives the most sets. If possible, get someone to videotape your opponents so that you can study the video before your next match. Or attend games where they are playing other teams so that you can check out individual players as well as the team style.

Remember the key players. When the US Women's Team plays Cuba, Russia, China, or Brazil, everyone spends a little extra time checking out the video. "These are the toughest kids on the block, and you have to be really prepared for these women," explains Endicott. "We watch and study their motions, then develop a mental picture of each opposing player. I visualize and lock into memory who the good blockers are, who the weak passers are, and who has the speed and agility. For me, as a setter, I can visualize what kinds of offense enhance our strength as a team."

Endicott remembers going into the 1991 World Cup in Japan and playing against Peru. The Peruvians had their setter in the middle blocking position, preparing to block the bigger hitters. "I knew we had to set the middle to take advantage of blocking this team offense," she says. "When we got there, we had imaged all of the strategies in advance, and it paid off. We took advantage of their weakness."

Rehearse in your mind. Suwara believes that to really understand and play the game of volleyball, athletes have to rehearse entire strategies in their minds before they get to the court. Even in the 1960s, before it was fashionable, Suwara used to visualize an entire game. "I would get relaxed in my own mind and go to my private volleyball court and imagine the athletes there," he says. "I would visualize the defense, our offense, and the set-ups. Even today I can recall one particular Russian, Valeri Kravchenko, a middle blocker who I would try to avoid. He was very tough. I would stay very high and keep the ball off the top of him. He was awesome, and I would always prepare for him in my mental rehearsal."

Visualize your actions. Before every match, Endicott and her teammates visualize specific plays that work against certain teams. She says that the advance mental practice training always pays off. "Anticipation is something you build on every day," she explains, "a skill that you can learn and

MENTAL MASTERS

Lori Endicott was a member of the 1992 and 1996 US Olympic Volleyball Teams. In 1990, she helped her team bring home the bronze medal at the World Championship. A former top-ranked player at the University of Nebraska in Lincoln, she has been playing volleyball since the late 1970s.

Rudy Suwara was assistant coach of the US Men's Olympic Volleyball Team in 1996. He competed in the Olympics in 1968 and 1972 and was a member of the winning Pan Am team.

Yoko Zetterlund played on the bronze-medal US Volleyball Team in the 1992 Olympics in Barcelona and on the women's Grand Prix tournament in 1993. She was a member of the 1996 US Olympic Team.

Mike Gaffaney played for UCLA all 4 years of his collegiate career and was a member of the national championship UCLA Bruin dynasty from 1981 to 1984.

enhance with practice. Volleyball is a sport of anticipation and expectation—knowing in advance who is going to set, who is going to tip, and who is going to spike."

TIPS FOR THE WHOLE TEAM

If anyone knows that the "whole is greater than the sum of its parts," it's Mike Gaffaney. A member of four national championship teams at UCLA (1981 to 1984), Gaffaney did not get all the minutes that he wanted, but enough to be a part of the dynasty. "When you have big guns on your team who are also Olympians, sometimes you have to spend time on the bench," he told me recently. "But I loved our program, and we had a strong team ethic, and that is what counts in this sport."

To be the stellar team contributor Gaffaney was, you'll want to follow these tips.

Keep your rhythm. Volleyball is 50-50: 50 percent mental and 50 percent physical, according to Olympian Zetterlund. She feels that the game is about rhythm and flow. "When our Olympic Team is struggling with passing, then we don't have flow and energy that is in sync with our game plan," she says. "That's when we get into trouble. Part of getting the team in flow is to move your feet and anticipate the correct body position. Anticipation of positioning gets you mentally prepared to hit the ball well and get the best possible shot."

Anticipate the ball. When I saw Zetterlund and her fellow athletes in action at the Russian Goodwill Games in 1994, I understood her notion of anticipation and physical and emotional awareness of ball movement. When Zetterlund practices imagery skill building, it is usually around the expectation and anticipation of where the ball is about to be hit. She suggests that if you can visualize that expectation, you are always going to be a half second ahead of the ball and ready for great defense.

Team play is the ticket. In the United States, the sport of volleyball is taking off on every level, says Endicott. "Coaches are getting better training and becoming much more scientific about the game," she says. "The team ethic of building a cohesive spirit is catching on in clubs and high schools across the nation. It is a lot more fun because kids are starting earlier and really learning the game. There is constant communication among the athletes and a mutual support system. It is much more about team play than just six individual egos diving for balls."

Gaffaney agrees. "In the sport of volleyball, at almost every level, a skilled, well-disciplined team will experience success far more than a team with gifted athletes but who do not work well as a team," he says.

Communicate, communicate, communicate. The best athletes are the ones who stay disciplined in their movements, are focused, and who communicate with one another on the court, says Endicott. She reminds volleyballers not to get frustrated with mistakes and not to dwell on a bad play. "Move ahead to the next play, expect the ball at all times—anticipate!" she says.

Redirect your rage. Endicott plays a more focused game when she is angry, because she channels her frustration and rage into some tough play. "The excitement in a volleyball game is contagious, so it had better be positive excitement and not the negative stuff. I'm intense, and I try to fire everyone up, but it can go both ways. When you are out of sync or out of focus, call a time-out and make substitutions. When things are not working well, it's important to have time to reassess. Talk to your teammates."

Keep your defense private. Brian Ivie is a rising star in Olympic volleyball. "Brian is an outstanding spiker and a great blocker," says his coach, Suwara. "He can analyze other teams' offense and set up an awesome defense to counter it. He is a great organizer on the court and has the uncanny ability to not give away his position. He is so skillful at disguising our defense that opponents have no idea what our game plan is."

Work together. Suwara is a true believer in mental training. He has contracted with sport psychologists to assist his Olympians with relaxation, imagery focus, and anticipation exercises. He encourages his athletes to listen to audiotape and review video in preparation for any competition. "I try and get our athletes to imagine they are doing each action perfectly," he says. "I want our team of six players to be in total flow—in sync with each other. I really believe that if a team is completely in a flow pattern, you don't have six players out there, you have seven (the players plus the team as a unit). And that's when exciting things start to happen on the court. The team is really a team."

SECRETS OF SUCCESS:
YOKO ZETTERLUND

Do It Until You Get It Right

Poor ball control in volleyball can be corrected by basic skill development, says Olympic volleyballer Yoko Zetterlund. Practice setting, spiking, passing, and returning—then practice some more. She also recommends lots of mental preparation to help correct flaws in play. Because volleyball is a physically demanding sport, she cross-trains, spending many hours a day on the track alternating sprints with longer distances.

COACHING IS CRITICAL

Suwara says the problem with elite volleyball players today is training time. "We don't get the kind of quality training and competition time that other countries have," he explains. "Our developmental programs are not yet strong, colleges are not pushing the sport, and when you do get elite players, they often go on the pro circuit." Times have changed since Suwara played in the late 1960s and early 1970s. He sees a whole new shift in the quality of players, and he now coaches athletes who come to the sport from basketball, track, and even gymnastics.

Team cohesiveness is crucial in this sport, but it is difficult to develop. Players come from all different disciplines and have many agendas. "You get athletes that are so gifted and talented and some who are not team players," says Suwara. "They are very independent and want to do their own thing. The countries that are dominating this sport are the ones with a strong team ethic. That takes lots of training and team building."

Suwara is a stickler for good team defense. He claims that if every athlete does his job, the whole team becomes an effective unit. "There is often a conflict because some of the athletes are very creative on the court. Blending our team is very hard," he explains. "You need to explore an individual's creativity on the court. An athlete like Dan Landry, a starting outside hitter on the National Team, will spot a play developing. He can go somewhere to make the play. Sometimes the ball falls between two people, in the 'ozone of responsibility,' and Danny will know exactly how and when to be there to get that ball."

A good coach must know the players and their strengths in this game and will diagnose a situation and know who is able to respond in the reflex situation. "As a coach, I need to push boundaries with some players. I need to encourage certain athletes to push the envelope to get those shots," says Suwara.

"We work with optometrists to improve eye awareness and coordination to better track moving objects," says Suwara. "We use a battery of tests to assess tracking in the visual field. When you look at an athlete like two-time Olympian Karch Kiraly, you see that he had phenomenal visual ability, depth perception, and peripheral vision. People like that see the holes in the blocking. They can read a defense, which can set a whole team in a positive motion.

SECRETS OF SUCCESS:
RUDY SUWARA

Work Hard, Play Hard

Volleyball is about speed and agility. Olympic volleyball coach Rudy Suwara cautions that to play the game at any level, you have to be physically fit. Jumping, bounding, strength training, and plenty of court time are what it takes to be good. Speed workouts to enhance reflexes and jumping are the best, says Suwara. Resistance and explosive training also help you prepare for the game.

"Volleyball has become more of a science," he says. "It is now a blend of the physical, the technical, and the visual preparation. The great athletes will spend time working on all three."

WORKSHEET: MENTAL TRAINING FOR VOLLEYBALL

Review these mental training techniques before your next few matches. Customize these tools to meet your individual goals and needs, then note what works for future competitions.

Use affirmations and self-talk. Practice these during training as well as competitions. Tell yourself during a tough match or workout, "I can do this." Don't allow negative thoughts such as "That other team looks awfully strong" or "I don't think I can make this return." If your team falls behind or you hit the ball out of bounds, tell yourself, "Stay calm; put it behind you." Choose a cue word or phrase such as "You can do it" to use in tough spots during the competition.

Breathe right. Practice full breathing regularly (see Chapter 4 for specific practice steps). Before your match, you may want to listen to a specific piece of music to practice relaxed, comfortable breathing. You might want to pair an image, such as making a powerful serve or return, with your breathing routine.

Meditate. Meditation prior to competition or practice will help you shut out the outside world and concentrate on your own game. You may choose a mantra such as Endicott's "Expect the ball; anticipate!" to repeat before and during the game to help you concentrate.

Relax. After hard workouts, practice progressive relaxation to relax your muscles. Establish your own relaxation routine with an audiotape. Practice a mini relaxation session, perhaps taking deep breaths or counting backward from 10, to calm yourself or relax overly tense muscles. Also, sit with teammates and have a group "quieting session." Let the team captain walk you through a visual strategy setting up various plays for on-court competition. By working together as a team in your mental practice, you will then react as a team in real time during court play.

Practice imagery and visualization. To begin guided imagery, identify how you view images by filling out the questionnaire on page 56. For imagery practice, watch film clips of pro competitions, which you can tape yourself from televised games or buy through the US Volleyball Association. You'll find a guided imagery program on page 240.

Consider other players. Volleyball is a team sport, so you need to visualize not only the opposing team but also your own teammates. Zetterlund's customized program includes watching videotapes of her team in action. This objective visual screening allows her to see the entire movement of her teammates and prepare for setting and spiking.

Visualize technique. Watch yourself serving, blocking the ball, spiking, and setting up the ball. Slow down your visualization, analyze your technique, and correct any errors in your style. Also, in volleyball, it's crucial to anticipate where the ball will land. This way, you can be ahead of the ball and ready to return it.

Build a victory image. See yourself and your teammates winning the last point that will carry the match. Feel the exhilaration, hear the spectators cheer, and watch yourself and your teammates jump into the air and thump each other on the backs in celebration. Enjoy that tired but exuberant feeling.

Use visual motor behavior rehearsal (VMBR). Visualize yourself in a competition; focus on enhancing your passing, serving, and returning techniques. Analyze your errors and mentally correct them, then mentally practice the right moves. While training, practice the corrected behavior. Before matches, imagine all the details and how you will meet challenges that might arise. Practice switching back and forth between a relaxed phase and a ready-to-win state of mind (see page 65 for specific steps). You could practice being relaxed and self-assured and confidently returning balls that fall into your zone of responsibility.

Have a precompetition routine. Anticipate, prepare for, and minimize as many distractions as possible. At the competition site, check out the surroundings, the spectators, and the noise. Check out each member of the opposing team. Thirty minutes before game time, move into your PTEZ, or perfect timing and energy zone. Practice relaxed breathing; visualize yourself serving, spiking, setting up, dealing with lost points or missed shots, scoring well, and ultimately winning the match. Tell yourself that you and your team will do well in this game. Do any precompetition rituals that make you more comfortable. For her ritual, Zetterlund likes to meet with her teammates to draw their energy together.

CHAPTER 20

Weight Training: Reach Your Power Summit

Once considered the domain of muscle-bound gym rats and users of questionable nutrients and other substances, weight training is being discovered by more and more people. Male and female athletes alike are taking up weight training, either as a cross-training activity or as a sport in itself. Young men and women are excited and see it as a helpful aid to sports involving short, explosive movements such as sprinting, high jumping, basketball, gymnastics, and discus throwing. Others take up weight training for its own merits or as part of a weight-control program. Performed properly, weight training is also a low-injury sport.

Some people who start out using weight training as part of their cross-training for other sports get interested in lifting competitions. World record setter and multiple medal holder Robin Byrd Goad left gymnastics at age 13, when she was noticed as a potential champion on the weight lifting circuit.

"When I was a gymnast, I spent time doing weight work. This was part of our injury prevention and strengthening techniques," she explains. "But I fooled everyone, including myself—and fell in love with the weight work. I achieved big gains with weight lifting very quickly and was ranked fifth in the nation at age 14. I was breaking all the stereotypical barriers for girls in weight lifting. I was this cute little gymnast breaking into the macho sport of weight lifting; it was really fun!"

FOR THOSE ABOUT TO LIFT

Whether training for personal satisfaction or for competition, mental practice will help you become a safer, stronger lifter. Byrd Goad, one of the leading weight lifters in the world, credits much of her success to mental practice and rehearsal. As a gymnast, she trained with imagery and visualization strategies. She also learned the discipline of training long hours, rehearsing routine after routine, and getting the muscle memory trained. Here are some mental training tips from Byrd Goad and other top lifters.

Enjoy your training. The most important element to remember in weight training, says Byrd Goad, is to enjoy the training process. Train with partners, both male and female. "Weight training and lifting are sociable," she says. "You set goals for yourself, but you can also compete against your buddies, pushing a little harder each day, stretching the envelope." Byrd Goad also suggests following a strength program—a scheduled training agenda.

Rehearse without lifting. John Coffee of the Coffee Gym outside Atlanta, head coach of the women's World Championship Team, and coach of the National Team, feels that seeing your weight in advance, or doing visual weight training, is very important. He will often have his athletes rehearse visually a particular weight sequence before a training session. "I have my athletes close their eyes and visualize a particular lift. I also get my athletes to ready themselves by doing some passive concentration exercises," he says. Passive concentration is focusing on the weight and the size of the lift without getting your energies invested heavily in the outcome. In other words, you go for the lift in your mind without feeling too much pressure to win.

Challenge yourself. All athletes have a natural desire to win and an affinity for achievement, says Olympic lifter Brian Jacob, who set five American records, and this holds true with weight training. There is an inherent challenge each day. That motivation gets you to push yourself harder, lifting a little more, so that your training partner doesn't beat you or simply so that you can improve your own performance. "I try to convey the message that weight training is something that comes over time," says

Jacob. "It isn't that difficult to get motivated in the weight room. You can always push the limits. You always have a challenge: to load more weight on the bar."

Visualize the right way. Byrd Goad, truly one of the toughest competitors around, works out with Jacob. She says that mental preparation is a big part of her training, even before she gets to the gym. "When I use visualization, I see myself using the proper technique and correcting that technique. To get ready for my big lifts, I do my mental rehearsal in the warmup room."

Follow your rituals. Byrd Goad has a preperformance ritual that she follows with precision and dedication. It is a ritual that allows for a steady stream of confidence and success in her sport. "I listen to my tape. The right music is very important to get me to that level of confidence," she says. "I listen to two songs, both by Van Halen from their *Standing on Top of the World* album. When I hear that music, I feel the fire, the competitive juices, and my aggression. Then I know it is time to wake up the nerve endings and go for it. I really start to believe in myself when I hear that music. I know that my hard training is done, the homework is complete, and now it is payoff time. I keep reminding myself that I'm strong, I'm in shape, and I have put in the hours."

Visualize feathers. Weight training is a sport that consultants are just beginning to understand with regard to mental practice. Most of the champion lifters explain that weight is just a figment of our imaginations. When we lift, we can believe that we are lifting the world. If you can visualize and mentally rehearse lifting a bed of feathers, your perception will be much different than if you visualize lifting lead.

Focus on the here and now. Byrd Goad visualizes herself doing the correct technique; she listens to her thoughts, and they are very clear. When she lifts, she does not think about the future but focuses on the present. "In the warmup room, I try not to get too psyched up," she says. "I know how to turn on the adrenaline and let it flow just before my big lift. I don't want that adrenaline turned on too soon, or I can lose my edge. I don't want to peak out before I'm ready to lift. I feel that I can turn it on like a key. I have it down to a science. I get very calm and relaxed right before I lift, and then I talk to my adrenaline and let it flow right before the moment of competition."

Let the past go. Jacob says that if you dwell on the past or think about a bad lift, you're in trouble. "When you snatch, you lift straight from the floor over your head all in one motion," he says. "This takes enormous concentration and inner strength to remember that you have the ability and talent to do this. The clean and jerk is done in two motions. First you lift to your chest from the floor and then from your chest to over your head. This is a different strategy and can require a different type of mental rehearsal."

Harness your anger. You can get frustrated during lifting. Byrd Goad says, "I sometimes get mad at myself when I'm not training well, and then the anger seems to turn around my attitude. I use anger to pump myself up. A few years ago my coach, John Coffee, would irritate me and say stuff that would set me off. I finally realized that John was manipulating the environment to bring out my anger and ultimately the best in my competitiveness. He knew the right buttons to push. . . . He was very respectful of my anger and knew how to tap into it productively."

MENTAL MASTERS

Robin Byrd Goad has competed in every World Championship every year since 1987 and set a world record in the snatch (in the 110-pound category) at 78 kilograms (171.6 pounds). Byrd Goad was the silver medalist in 1987, 1988, 1992, and 1993. She has also brought home the gold from the Olympic Festival every year since 1989. She competed in Sydney in the first-ever women's Olympic team in the 48-kilogram weight class and finished fifth.

John Coffee trains many world-renowned weight lifters in the Coffee Gym outside Atlanta. Coffee has been head coach of the women's World Championship Team since 1991 and the National Team coach since 1980. He coaches Robin Byrd Goad, Sibby Flowers, Coleen Coley, Christy Byrd, Jane Camp, and Lynn Stoessel.

Brian Jacob placed 18th in the Olympics in 1992 with a personal record of 122.5 kilograms (269.5 pounds) in the snatch event and 150 kilos (330 pounds) in the clean and jerk competition. He set five American records and finished 11th in the Australian World Championship in 1991. He placed ninth in the 1996 Olympics.

Give yourself a break. Byrd Goad trains 6 days a week, 2 hours a day. She understands that her body needs a light day occasionally between heavy lifting days. When she feels fatigue setting in, she doesn't push it. She knows that there's usually a reason for the fatigue. She also has a number of other interests away from the weight room, including hiking, skiing, and even hand quilting. The quilting is for relaxation. Choose your own restful activity to give yourself some time off from the lifting routine.

HOW CHAMPIONS PREPARE TO COMPETE

If you decide to enter competition or if weight lifting is your primary sport, you may want to modify your approach to better meet the higher demands. Here's how.

Find a good coach. One important part of learning the sport of weight lifting is getting hooked up with a qualified coach, says Coffee. You need to have the right physiological and psychological makeup before you begin. Most important, you need a coach who understands the sport and knows the potential dangers—someone you can trust. He suggests that athletes under age 12 (with the exception of highly developed preteens) not engage in weight training. "You don't want to push kids too early, both from a physiological and developmental perspective as well as an emotional one. In general, if you have an athlete with some prior training, you can move into weight work slowly and do body buildups on machines. But when you get to the serious free weights, then you have to be careful. And you must be coached by a competent professional."

Concentrate on positive images. Jacob focuses on positives rather than negatives when he lifts. He is constantly asking himself, "What do I have to do to make this a successful lift?" He tries to keep his focus on positive imagery. "The lifts that I do make are the ones with positive images in my head," he says. Jacob is not one to dwell on doubt, but he obsesses about the right posture and the correct form and about keeping his positive thoughts in sync with the weight he wants to clear. "If I keep my back tight, I'm going to make the lift. My experience has been that when I am trying to fix something, I don't succeed. I have three attempts to make a lift, and I need to think that I'm going to make it each time."

Take care not to overpsych. With weight lifting, as in other explosive sports, it doesn't do any good to get psyched too far in advance, according to Byrd Goad. Athletes need to know their pace, visualizing themselves on the

------

SECRETS OF SUCCESS:
ROBIN BYRD GOAD

Slow and Easy Does It

When you first start training, don't move too fast, cautions top lifter Robin Byrd Goad. Progressing slowly and building a base are the safest ways to learn the sport. Research with weight lifters suggests that you should be age 13 or 14 before you start pumping iron. You need a good strength training coach, someone who knows the sport. Working all aspects of the body is important, and finding the balance with your strengths and weaknesses is a primary concern.

Byrd Goad trains in the gym by pulling deadlift shrugs. These are assistance exercises, and they help in strengthening parts of the body. She also does front squats and back squats. Military presses, abdominal work, reverse situps and Rumanian deadlifts are all part of her vocabulary. She suggests finding a qualified coach and working out with a team or group. Spotting is essential, not only for safety but for moral support as well.

Weight lifting is just starting to come into its own, says Byrd Goad. Today there are approximately 500 women and 1,500 men registered as competitive weight lifters. For women, it was initiated as an Olympic sport in Sydney.

------

platform, seeing and feeling the arena, imagining the competition, and becoming more familiar with the surroundings. Byrd Goad experiences her sport as an athlete would skiing, playing basketball, or any other major competition. You need to get acclimated and visualize the venue before you get there.

Don't overfocus. Coffee is quick to remind his athletes that weight training must be fun, and there has to be joyfulness in each lift. "You have to be mentally focused, but in the same breath you have to be very loose," he says. "You don't want to be too focused or too intense. There is a certain personality that allows you to progress and be a champion in this sport." In big-time competitions, Coffee will try to distract an athlete if it is appropriate. He will try to get a competitor to loosen up by telling a funny story so that he has a positive distraction.

A NEW LOOK TO WEIGHT TRAINING

With the proliferation of funding of women's athletics because of Title IX and so many superb female athletes in basketball, soccer, softball, and tennis, there is a whole new quality of US athlete emerging. "I see US women getting into the sport and ladies from all over the world lifting weights and competing," says Coffee. Many of his current athletes come from sports such as gymnastics, track and field, softball, and basketball.

"I have an interest in seeing women develop their strength and physiology," says Coffee. "Women are different psychologically; they have a different style of competitive behavior. I can work with a talented woman

SECRETS OF SUCCESS: BRIAN JACOB

Getting a Lift from Social Support

Olympic lifter Brian Jacob, who set five American records, works out 5 days a week, training for a total of 20 hours. He reminds beginning lifters that motivation, patience, and much hard work are the ingredients for strong outcomes. "It takes a long time, sometimes 5 years of hard training, to see any big-time results," he says. "It's not a glamour event."

Jacob does not believe in machines—no pulleys, cables, or pneumatic systems for this guy—just free weights. He uses assistance exercises to help physically and emotionally. "We do partial movements, pulling from the floor, and squats to enhance performance and to get stronger." He also recommends training with a partner, and he trains with three to six people in the gym. "I have never seen people who train by themselves improve as much as those who train with a team," he says. "We all have up and down days, but with a group, somebody is usually having an up day, and that gets transmitted so that we motivate each other."

athlete in 6 months and make her a champion. With men it might take 5 years." Weight lifting competition can offer opportunities into the masters age range, Coffee notes. One of the athletes he has trained is Jane Black, who won a title in the masters category at age 42.

Women have evolved culturally in the sport of weight lifting, says Coffee, and there's no longer a masculine stigma attached to women who lift weights. "Today, it is a different cultural norm," he says. "Women want to be trim and toned. Body styles have changed, and so people in general are looking different. Women want to be stronger, more assertive, and efficient and carry heavier loads, work harder, and hold a different societal ethic."

Weight lifting has deep historical roots, says Coffee. Back in the 1930s and 1940s, strength magazines encouraged women to lift to get in shape. In the 1950s, it was a sport with a small but prestigious following. Hollywood starlets such as Jayne Mansfield and Marilyn Monroe lifted weights so that they could stay fit and toned. Today, Coffee sees the sport emerging in a different way. "I travel all over the world with these great women athletes. I love going to all these foreign nations and seeing the status, the prestige, and the unique talent that the sport is attracting."

WORKSHEET: MENTAL TRAINING
FOR WEIGHT TRAINING

Review these mental training techniques before your next lifting session. You'll want to customize these tools to meet your own goals and needs and take note of what images or techniques work best for you.

Use affirmations and self-talk. Practice these during training as well as during competition. Tell yourself during a tough workout or competition, "I can do this." Don't allow negative thoughts such as "Those other lifters look awfully strong" or "I don't think I can make this lift." If you botch a lift, put it behind you. Choose a cue word or phrase such as "You can do it" to use while you are lifting.

Breathe right. Practice full breathing regularly (see Chapter 4 for specific practice steps). Before your competition or workout, you may want to listen to a specific piece of music to practice relaxed, comfortable breathing. You might want to pair an image, such as making a successful lift, with your breathing routine. As you lift, it is important to inhale fully, being sure never to hold your breath. Holding your breath serves only to tighten and constrain various muscle groups. Then exhale gently at the end of your lift and allow your lungs to be free of excess air as you complete your maneuver.

Meditate. Meditation while lifting will help you shut out the outside world and concentrate on your own performance. You might choose a mantra such as Byrd Goad's "I'm strong; I'm in shape" to repeat while lifting to help you concentrate and stay relaxed.

Relax. After hard workouts, practice progressive relaxation to relax your muscles. Establish your own relaxation routine with an audiotape. Practice a mini relaxation session, perhaps using deep breaths or counting backward from 10 to calm yourself or relax overly tense muscles just before a lift. You can also use what is called differential relaxation, learning to control various muscle groups so you can relax the ones you aren't using to lift, even during competitions.

Practice imagery and visualization. For imagery practice, watch lifting competitions on television or have someone videotape you lifting. To begin guided imagery, identify how you view images by filling out the questionnaire on page 56. In your mind, watch yourself during a lifting session, slow down your visualization, and correct any mistakes you see in your technique. You'll find a guided imagery program on page 240.

Consider your opponent. Jacob likes to visualize an opponent and then forget he exists. He knows the competition, but ultimately he knows "it is up to me and my training and mental toughness to hit the weight I have prepared for. No other competitor will impact my performance. I am my best opponent and my worst opponent, depending on my mental game that day."

Visualize technique. The mental training program Byrd Goad uses allows her to see and feel the proper weight lifting technique. As a world record holder in the 110-pound division, Byrd Goad likes to visualize the weight and, more important, her approach to the weight. With the proper technique, she points out, anyone can do weight training and competitive lifting.

Build a victory image. This is a sport that both men and women are doing more of and is part of a cross-training regimen for nearly all competitive sports. If it's not your primary sport, enjoy your weight work as time away from your competitive sport. If you're a competitive lifter, develop an image of an explosive, powerful lift and imagine the feelings that accompany a successful lift.

Use visual motor behavior rehearsal (VMBR). Visualize yourself lifting; focus on enhancing your technique and analyzing and mentally correcting errors. While training, practice the corrected behavior. Before lifting, imagine all the details and how you will meet challenges as they arise, such as pain or tightness, a sense of fatigue, or a strained or pulled muscle. Practice switching back and forth between a relaxed phase and a ready-to-win state of mind (see page 65 for specific steps).

Have a precompetition routine. Anticipate, prepare for, and minimize as many distractions as possible. At the competition site, check out the surroundings, the crowd, and the noise. Look around to see who your competitors are. Thirty minutes before your event, move into your PTEZ, or perfect timing and energy zone. Practice relaxed breathing. Visualize yourself competing and finishing strongly. Tell yourself that you will do well in this competition or workout. Do any precompetition rituals that make you more comfortable. Byrd Goad is the ultimate competitor, but she likes to hear or tell a joke before she competes. This is her ritual for preparation in a major competition.

CHAPTER 21

Pentathlon: The Ultimate in Cross-Training

Few sports test the body and challenge the emotions like the modern pentathlon. As Pernille Svarre, the Danish gold medalist from the 2001 World Championships and Sydney Olympian says, "It takes everything you have, in five disciplines, all in one day. You can't just show up unprepared, tired, or not focused in this sport."

For the uninitiated, the pentathlon is a backbreaking multihour event that dares competitors to perform five sports with professional skill, beginning with riflery, and moving on to fencing, a 200-meter swim, equestrian riding and jumping, and finally a 3000-meter cross-country run. All in one day. As Roderick Martin, vice president for the Modern Pentathlon Federation, says, "The sport demands that you call up all of your focused energy from every pore in your body so that you can perform at the highest emotional level."

To train in the pentathlon is a call for multiple disciplines. It is a summoning of an enormous amount of discipline and inner focus, according to Chad Senior. He and teammate at the world championships, Eli Bremer, a recent graduate of the Air Force Academy, believe that the mental side of the sport is probably the toughest. According to Bremer, "It is the vision and perseverance and courage to get up each morning and know that you will be trying to perform efficiently at each venue. This means allocation of time and energy to each sport without stressing your system too hard. It's a real balancing act."

Typically, pentathlon athletes come from running backgrounds; some are former swimmers who also ran track and cross country. Some come to the sport as outstanding fencers. The demands of time and resources are very tough. Often athletes will come from the military, which supports a very strong pentathlon training program. But the sport does nurture the best and the brightest.

ANYTHING CAN HAPPEN

Perhaps the biggest mental trick in preparing for the pentathlon is preparing for anything. With five events to worry about, an athlete must be prepared for five completely different sets of variables. If your gun jams, your fencing fails, your swimming goes awry, your horse falters, or you experience leg problems, you must be prepared. Svarre says it best: "You have to be ready for the unexpected."

Emily deRiel, who gave a historic pentathlon performance in September 2000 in Sydney, when she won the silver medal, agrees.

"With so many events and so many unknowns, there's a lot that can go wrong in pentathlon," says deRiel, a Yale graduate who can break down the mental side of pentathlons with the same insight she brought to her studies. "You have to practice being flexible."

Before and during competitions, deRiel reassures herself that she is the driving force behind how she does, not her equipment or her horse. "I didn't panic if things went wrong," she says. "Before the shoot in the Olympics, for instance, I couldn't find my receipt without which I couldn't pick up my gun—due to the strict gun regulations in Australia, they were kept locked up, and we only had access to them during practice or the competition itself. I could have gotten worked up into a panic, which would have negatively impacted my shoot. Instead, I made myself stay calm, telling myself it would work out, and sure enough, our team manager had taken the receipt out of my bag on his own and had picked up my gun for me."

To help cut down on the potential for mistakes and confusions, deRiel makes a few suggestions on how to prepare for an event.

Don't rush yourself the morning of a competition. "Take time packing the night before; it can be a kind of ritual unto itself," she says.

"You don't want to be running around the morning of a competition looking for something. First, you might forget things, and second, you'll get anxious and that might set the tone for the day."

MENTAL MASTERS

Pernille Svarre competed in 20 World Championships from the beginning in 1981 to 2001. She won a silver medal in 1984, team bronze in 1994 and 1995, and gold in 2000. And she got to fulfill her ultimate dream: She took part in the first Olympic Games of Women's Modern Pentathlon in Sydney 2000.

Vahktang Jagorachvili has a career that goes back to the mid-1970s. He won gold at junior worlds in 1985. He then took first place at the Goodwill Games of 1986 in Moscow. The next win was huge. Competing for the Soviet Union from the Republic of Georgia, Jagorachvili took the Olympic bronze medal in the 1988 Seoul Olympics. He competed again in the 1996 games. He competed for the United States as a US Olympian in Athens in 2004 at the age of 40.

Emily deRiel graduated from Yale in 1996 and then went to Oxford as a Rhodes scholar and earned a degree in English literature. In between her studies, she found time to train and make the first women's Olympic team in pentathlon in Sydney 2000. She won the silver medal in Sydney at this historic event.

Anita Allen is a 2000 graduate of West Point and won the biggest competition of her life in Santo Domingo in August 2003 by winning the gold medal at the Pan Am Games. The win gave her an automatic berth for being a member of the US Olympic team in Athens 2004.

Kate Allenby competed for the United Kingdom in Sydney and won the bronze medal. Earlier in her career, she won gold at the 1993 Junior World Championships, a 1997 gold at the Europeans, World Cup gold, and bronze at the World Championships in 2003.

Know your eating and drinking needs. I used to drink coffee or have a caffeinated PowerGel before and during the fence, as well as eat a banana or a power bar," she says. "You don't want to run out of steam before the end of the day, nor do you want to feel too full for the swim, for instance. It's very important to stay hydrated since it's such a long day, and with the run being the final event, dehydration can really take its toll there."

Get a good night's sleep two nights before a competition. "This is a general rule; you never know if you'll have insomnia the night before. People say it's the sleep two nights before that's most important anyway. I find that adrenaline can get you pretty far, so don't panic if you didn't sleep well."

Be the one working the hardest. "There were some training sessions that I would just have to try to get through because I was feeling tired or worn out. Usually, though, I tried to always find something to work on. During track workouts, I would try to imagine how I would feel in the last 1000 meters of the race, and I would work that much harder to make those last 1000 meters better. Or I would think while swimming about how it would feel to be just behind a competitor and how I would want to have the strength to move up and pass them. That helped to get me going when I felt like coasting."

KEEPING YOUR HEAD IN THE GAMES

To stay focused during the pentathlon, deRiel offers a number of strategies. Here are her top suggestions.

Balance rest with keeping active and alert. You want to save your legs as much as possible during a 10-hour competition, but there is also a danger of getting *too* mellow and starting to feel drowsy, deRiel says. If that happens, "it can get hard to get yourself going again," she says. "Pay attention to your body, and if you feel yourself getting sleepy or tightening up, move around, stretch, make yourself laugh, and wake yourself up."

Relax. While different athletes relax differently, deRiel suggests using humor. "Especially during the shoot, I would tell jokes to myself to break the tension," she says. "Or I would think of funny lines from the *Simpsons* or *Saturday Night Live* or from the David Sedaris books to make me smile and to help me lighten up."

Focus on the present event or challenge. Once an event is over, let it be over, deRiel says. "For me, the fence was always difficult, so I had to concentrate on that while I was actually fencing each bout. As soon as we moved on to the swim, I put the fence behind me, no matter how I had done, and focused on what I had to do in the swim. Then the ride and the run. With such a long competition day, it's dangerous to think too far ahead or dwell on the mistakes you made earlier."

Act as you want to feel. DeRiel learned this lesson just before the 2000 Olympics. "It's amazing how the body can influence the mind to feel ways it didn't before," she says. "I would smile, stand up straight, move confidently, and I actually felt better—happier, less nervous." On the day of an event, deRiel also tries to focus on enjoying the day itself rather than fixating on winning or losing. "Not only did I perform better, but even if I hadn't, I would have had a better time doing it, so it was win-win," she says.

Develop rituals. "With an event like shooting where so much is mental, you need a way for your body to pick up some of the slack so you don't have to think about every little thing," deRiel says. If you have a routine, "you feel in familiar territory no matter where you are shooting." Before shooting, deRiel's routine goes something like this: Look down at your toes. Breathe deep. Adjust your fingers on the grip of the gun while it's resting on the table. Then find a spot on the floor slightly ahead of your feet in the direction of the target and focus on that. "I would feel a wave of relaxation start at the top of my head and flow down, another deep breath, raise the gun past the target, lower it, and gradually pull the trigger back," she says. "If I got distracted or felt rushed, I'd stop and start over again."

Of course, sometimes patently absurd events occur that are well beyond the realm of planning. An extreme example of this happened to Vahktang Jagorachvili, the old wise man of cross-training and one of the preeminent modern pentathlon athletes in the world (he won the gold in the 2003 Pan Am Games, automatically earning a spot on the US Olympic Team in Athens).

"I handle competition very well because I know that you don't have control over all of the world; stuff happens." Jagorachvili was referring to an event that we both shared in July 2003 in Pesaro, Italy, at the World Championships. During the final event of the daylong competition, the 3000-meter run, two local Italian men got into a street fight and stabbed each other. They both lay bleeding in the street; in fact, right in the middle of the race course for the event. Police and ambulances had to intervene, and the race was stopped. It was, to say the least, surreal.

I was standing just a few feet from Jagorachvili when the chaos broke out. The competition had to be postponed for 40 minutes, and many athletes were upset, cooling down, and losing their edge. He looked at me; and we both started laughing. "I just knew it was crazy, some random event that I had no control over . . . so I just started to laugh, relax, stretch out, and know that my start time would be delayed. To get upset and lose my focus would be stupid and counterproductive," he said. "Sometimes the weirdest things happen in

SECRETS OF SUCCESS: ANITA ALLEN

Shooting: "I use visualization in between shots during practice. On the way to an event, I will sit and relax and clear my head, get centered, and calm myself. In competition, I visualize before the event. I use key words to structure my thoughts and calm myself."

Fencing: "On the day of competition, I do a warmup that makes me feel good, a warmup that builds my confidence. I prepare in my mind ahead of time, and then it becomes automatic. Also, in fencing, there is a lot of noise, a lot of high stress, so I try to keep other people out of it and keep the distractions out."

Swimming: "I rehearse the swim mentally until I feel that I have already been there. I visualize my turns, hitting the wall, and releasing from the wall. I'm so relaxed in the water from my earlier preparation that it seems automatic."

Equestrian: "Riding is something I have to work at, so on the day of competition, I memorize and blueprint the course. I use positive affirmations with my horse, especially if I get a refusal (when a horse balks at a jump and you have to reenter the course). I know what the backup plan is if this happens."

Running: "I'm confident and strong. I firmly believe that I'm as strong as my mind allows me to be. I need to be mentally prepared at all times. The race is 3000 meters, and I break it down into 1000-meter pieces and visualize each element of the race. That way I know my breathing, my tempo, my internal pace clock."

life, and you must just let go and not have total need for control; allow things to be as they are; that is my training and competition mentality at all times."

When Jagorachvili competes, he is very focused. "I have a bubble around me—I always go with the flow; I am very patient; I don't get worried too much, but I maintain my concentration and focus at all times." He also notes that it is important to release steam and stress when you have to. "I will go release my tension or my anxieties, but I do it privately. I do get emotional, but I don't blame anyone. I know myself so well that I coach myself, so it is natural. I know my heart rate. I know my redline areas like a Ferrari. I don't push the envelope and burn out the engine. So I know my internal tachometer, my equilibrium; I know the tipping point; I know how far I can push the machinery, both mentally and physically. I was trained in the Soviet system as a child, so there are certain barometers that you learn early on."

DEALING WITH PERSONAL TRAGEDY

Right before the 2003 Pan Am Games, Anita Allen faced what may be the hardest obstacle any athlete has to overcome: the death of a loved one. In this case, it was Leif E. Nott, a friend and former classmate of Allen's at the US Military Academy at West Point, New York. Leif, a first lieutenant in the army, was killed in Iraq just days before.

"August 3 was a nightmare for me," she says. "I found out that my best friend in the whole world, Leif Nott, had been killed in Iraq; it was devastating," she told me. "I had to prepare for my competition on August 11, and it was one of the all-time lows in my life. I was in such pain, I had an injury, and then my friend was shot in a firefight in Baghdad. It was horrendous. I thought about quitting the sport and just going home. But many of my West Point classmates were e-mailing me from the front lines in Iraq and giving me tons of emotional support; this helped me gain the courage to continue and then to compete."

Making things harder was the knowledge that other classmates were fighting the war while Allen was safe and competing in a sports event. "My entire class of 2000 at West Point was all very close," she says, "so I felt guilty about being in a safe, elite-athlete, cozy environment, when they were putting their lives on the line. I guess I had to process a lot of survivor guilt as well."

To work against her anger and guilt, Allen "just sort of let go psychologically" and focused on the event at hand. "During the competition, I knew that

SECRETS OF SUCCESS: KATE ALLENBY

Aussie-born and England-raised Kate Allenby has medaled in many of the pentathlon's biggest events, including a gold in 1993 at the Junior World Championships, a 1997 gold at the Europeans, World Cup gold, and Olympic bronze in Sydney, and then the World Championship bronze in 2003. Here are her tips for all the events.

Shooting: "This is the one I struggle with. I need to calm myself before shooting; I find it very stressful. I went to a hypnotherapist. He actually got me to fall into a trancelike sleep state before shooting; it keeps me very focused before shooting. I stare at one spot; I get tired and sleepy, but I stay alert. The hypnotic state keeps my heart rate low and my energy high and focused. You have to remember to count to three to wake up, and then I can move to the next event."

Fencing: "This one is a bit easier for me. I use the image of Maurice Green, the world class sprinter, before I fence. I growl, I say out loud, 'This is my space, this is my territory, you are coming to fence me; don't take over my space.' I do this little dance to psych myself up; this is my space, this is my area. My colleague and fellow Olympian Linford Christie (the prominent sprinter) was the same way. He would slam into people, he would own his lane before he did his 100-meter race. I'm very focused; I'm very aggressive; I feel on top of it. Sometimes I use video for fencing, and the visual feedback is very helpful."

I just had to go out there and get the job done," she says. "It was such a release of all the emotions, I just needed to go out and channel all that energy."

In a display of human perseverance, Allen went on to win the gold medal and qualify for the Olympics in Athens.

WORKSHEET: MENTAL TRAINING
FOR MULTISPORT AND PENTATHLON

Most people are not pentathletes, but many recreational athletes are turning to multiple sports for cross-training, to keep fresh, and to have fun.

Swimming: "I use visualization a lot for my swim event. I swim the race in my head; I visualize each turn; I feel each stride; I feel myself stretching out. During training, I do not use visualization, only in competition. Once again its *me* and my lane and my race. In swimming, I find that an under-water camera is helpful for stroke feedback and correction."

Equestrian: "I always walk the course in my head, in advance of the event. I go through the course and pace the distances in my head. I count my strides, and I measure my strides in my head. In pentathlon, you get random draws on horses. So there is an unpredictable variable in the ride: the size of the horse, its personality, and its temperament. I try and keep the horse alert as I go through checkpoints in my head. It's very important to do practice sessions before the event. If I don't like a horse, then I try and do my best not to let the horse know it. You have to feel the energy of the horse, its kinesthetic, and then adjust yourself."

Running: "I really hate running, but I have to deal with it. Since I'm not gifted or talented in running, I have to train hard. In warmups, I stay away from teammates so that I don't feel intimidated and negative. I want to be positive with my run event, and I need to overcome negativity. I go out at a good pace, but I don't get panicked; I have to make adjustments. I have to self-talk all the time to stay with a good pace as a nongifted runner."

Review the following recommendations and tailor these tips to your training.

All of us can benefit from mental training strategies, but take a look at how these techniques fit your objectives and goals.

Use affirmations and self-talk. Practice self-talk and positive affirmations during each of your warmups, your workouts, and after you finish— as you stretch and cool down. By telling yourself to relax, you can actually benefit from these affirmations.

Use positive images, and don't let negative thoughts creep into your mind. Even if one of your sports is difficult and strenuous, remind yourself of the positive imagery that you experienced during a pleasant workout.

Cue yourself to a positive image when you feel negative energy or fatigue emerging.

Before each event, for example in pentathlon, say the following: "I can shoot with great accuracy and steady hand. I can fence with strong and able legs. I can swim with enormous speed and stamina. I can ride and jump with ease. I can run swiftly and flawlessly."

Breathe right. Practice full and complete body breathing to get the most out of all of your sports (see Chapter 4 for specific practice steps). Breathe before and during all of the five events. Remember, breathing is the source of muscle relaxation and fluid motion. Use your breath when you shoot, fence, swim, ride, and run. It is the anchor for each of your mental training cues.

Breathing fully and completely will give you positive and productive energy and help you conserve energy for a long, long day of competition.

Meditate. This is very important, especially for long, hard, enduring multisport competitions. As silver medalist deRiel has noted, each event in pentathlon is separate and requires different types of emotional focus. Meditation helps you relax, calm your muscles, breathe appropriately, and achieve your individual motor tasks.

Practice imagery and visualization. Imagery is important in all sports, but especially when moving from one to another in a daylong or multiday competition. As Pan American Champion and Olympian, Allen has observed, "Imagery can assist with balance, focus, and concentration in each event." Use visualization to prepare for each event before you get there. The outcomes will be greatly improved.

Building a victory image. Since multisport events like pentathlon require intense physical and emotional energy, use imagery and the vision of victory to build strength for each venue.

CHAPTER 22

A Mental Practice Formula
for Any Sport

Regardless of your sport or the level of competition, mental practice can help you attain peak performance. No matter if you are a weekend warrior or a world-class athlete, using mental practice with the proper imagery and visualization will let you improve your response to whatever athletic challenge lies before you. And having a supportive coach, teacher, or mentor can assist that process enormously as we learned from previous chapters.

Although some athletes have very specific and personalized formulas for achieving the optimum mental state of preparation, there are basics that all of us can follow. Proper breathing and relaxation before a competitive event are mandatory. We also know that having confidence and a sense of well-being and feeling tuned up are all part of the preathletic preparation.

THE NUTS AND BOLTS OF MENTAL PRACTICE

Here are the basic principles of a customized mental training program, which you can adapt to fit your sport and your needs and desires.

Set goals. It's a trite but true saying that if you don't know where you're going, you'll never get there. You need to decide what you want to accomplish and plan your training accordingly. Janet Evans, the great Olympic champion, believes that whether you are an Olympian or a recreational athlete, you have to set your goals high and train hard. Olympic pentathlete and coach Vahktang Jagorachvili believes that solid planning is important in any mental practice program. He is thorough and precise about goal setting for the athletes he coaches, some of whom check in by phone, fax, or e-mail. He coaches a full gamut of competitive athletes ranging from high school to masters level, and he constantly reminds them to visualize their goals.

WRITE DOWN HERE WHAT WORKS FOR YOU.

_____

_____

_____

Use a verbal cue. Many athletes use cognitive mental training in their programs, both in training and in competition. Marathoner Benji Durden uses the mantra "I'm okay, I'm all right, and I'm doing fine." This saying, or verbal reinforcer, reminds Durden to take it easy during the stressful periods of the marathon. "Know thyself," he says. "When the going gets tough at the 20-mile mark, learn to use verbal cues or reminders that help you get through the Wall (that sense of doom and feeling of fatigue) or other times when fatigue sets in." These are cues that all of us can use during competition, but we have to first practice them in training.

WRITE DOWN HERE WHAT WORKS FOR YOU.

_____

_____

_____

Focus on the positive. Any top-level athlete will tell you that you can be your own worst enemy. If you think you're going to hit a pop fly, chances are that you will. If you think you're going to slow down while running up the big hill ahead, chances are that you will. Top-ranked pentathlete Chad Senior is a strong believer in mental practice and strength. He gets quite anxious before competitions and concentrates on converting that adrenaline to positive thoughts or emotions. He tries to remember that even though he is racing right on the edge, he must stay focused and not dwell on a potential negative. For any sport, think positively and keep telling yourself that you can do it.

WRITE DOWN HERE WHAT WORKS FOR YOU.

_____

_____

_____

Build in relaxation time. All work and no relaxation results in an overtrained athlete. Runner Maria Mutola, four-time Olympian and gold medalist in the 800 meters, includes a lot of rest in her training program. Before any meet, whether an all-comers or the Olympics, she takes 6 hours before the start to rest and mentally prepare for the competition. Her rest and relaxation is just one component of her mental rehearsal strategy. It's important for you to build rest into your training schedule to allow yourself to recuperate both mentally and physically.

WRITE DOWN HERE WHAT WORKS FOR YOU.

_____

_____

_____

Find the right tension level. In many sports, it's crucial to stay relaxed at the right moment. In tennis, for example, the most important element to learning this relaxation response is to hit hard and with passion, but learn to let down after each point. Tennis coach and sport mentor, Nick Bollettieri, known as the mental training expert in the tennis world, for example, actually measures heart rate between points. He emphasizes that your heart rate should be up during the heat of competition, but immediately following a point (regardless of who made the point), you must disengage, relax, and let your heart rate return to resting baseline. The closer you get to this relaxation response, the better conditioned mentally and physically you will be. The same holds true for many other sports. Identify when you need to be relaxed, and consciously work on relaxing at those times.

WRITE DOWN HERE WHAT WORKS FOR YOU.

_____

_____

_____

Take a look at your opponents. In just about any sport, you have to know the competition along with their strengths and weaknesses. You should visualize yourself competing, visualize all the other competitors, and visualize yourself finishing and winning, says Mutola. Study the venue. Whether you're participating in a triathlon or playing a soccer match, it's crucial that you're aware of the details of the place you're going to compete. Be aware of course markers or any idiosyncrasies of a race course. Mountain biking can be totally unpredictable, for instance, with many tough turns and rugged terrain. To predict the unpredictable and stay calm and focused, says John Tomac, you must run the course in your mind, visually rehearsing all the potential problems. That is the only way he will start a race, and it is also how he converts anxiety and jitters to positive and healthy race energy.

WRITE DOWN HERE WHAT WORKS FOR YOU.

_____

_____

_____

Visualize proper techniques. Diann Roffe-Steinrotter, a two-time Olympian and gold medalist in skiing, recommends not only seeing your imagery in a visual sense but also feeling it. Each sport has its specific moves: how you grip your golf club, how you kick the soccer ball, how you flick your wrists on a jump shot. You can be a powerful and well-trained athlete, but incorrect technique can pull your performance well below your capabilities. Top weight lifter Robin Byrd Goad concentrates on visualizing the proper weight lifting technique. As a world-record setter in the 110-pound division, Byrd Goad likes to visualize not only the weight itself, but also her approach to the weight.

WRITE DOWN HERE WHAT WORKS FOR YOU.

_____

_____

_____

Imagine coping with extremes. When preparing for your competition, you have to visualize the entire package, says Leann Warren, a former Olympic track star turned cycling champion. This means seeing, feeling, and hearing the weather, your conditioning (including fatigue), and the contours of the course. To be a great athlete, you have to know your boundaries, both in terms of energy output and fatigue levels, says Warren. Imagine yourself after 4 hours of riding. Imagine that fatigue level. Now crank yourself up by imagining what you feel like on a beautiful sunny day when you are starting out fresh with lots of energy. Those are the types of extremes that you have to practice in your imagery work, no matter what your sport.

WRITE DOWN HERE WHAT WORKS FOR YOU.

_____

_____

_____

Break out the videotape. In just about any sport, you'll benefit from a videotape of yourself in action, whether in training or in a race or competition. If you don't have a video camera, try to borrow or rent one. Yoko Zetterlund, an Olympic bronze-medal volleyball player, watches videotapes of herself as well as her whole team in action. This objective visual screening allows her to see each movement she makes and how individual team members move and prepare for setting and spiking.

WRITE DOWN HERE WHAT WORKS FOR YOU.

_____

_____

_____

See yourself winning. Build a mental image of yourself crossing the finish line, celebrating with your teammates after a big win, or turning to see your name at the top of the scoreboard. Olympic swimmer and multiple gold-medal winner Susie O'Neil visualizes all of her races and always prepares by seeing herself win. She is so focused about her mental preparation that she does not stop her training until she experiences the win in her mind's eye. That is her cue that she is ready to compete. She suggests that athletes practice their imagery as a team as well as by themselves. She feels that the collective energy of the team can set off a series of positive events. O'Neil rarely loses a race in the pool, and she never loses one in her mind.

WRITE DOWN HERE WHAT WORKS FOR YOU.

_____

_____

_____

Maintain cool under pressure. Every event brings some pressure, and top tennis player Andy Roddick (winner of the 2003 US Open) believes that a customized training program is all about learning to focus under pressure. He practices how to handle tension, pressure, and fatigue, both in his mind and on the court. He stays in the present, reminding himself to stay calm and relaxed no matter what the score is. His training agenda deals with winning and not getting there with too much ease. If he loses his edge or isn't focused, he tends to let his concentration lapse. For many sports, imagery practice includes balancing the highs and lows. This includes verbal cues and reminders such as "Get over that bad move." You need to concentrate on your sport; and if you make a mistake, move on and don't dwell on it.

WRITE DOWN HERE WHAT WORKS FOR YOU.

_____

_____

_____

Make your emotions work for you. Byrd Goad also believes in the emotion of anger. For many athletes, tuning into your own source of anger and channeling it can be very productive when competing. Byrd Goad knows herself and knows the mental strategies of her coach, John Coffee, of the Coffee Gym outside Atlanta, head coach of the Women's World Championship Team and coach of the National Team. According to Byrd Goad, "John manipulates the environment to bring out the anger in me so that I can be at my peak performance. It usually works very well." Whether a vision of passion, anger, or tranquility, find the right imagery button to push for yourself.

WRITE DOWN HERE WHAT WORKS FOR YOU.

_____

_____

_____

Develop your own rituals. Some athletes have special rituals that they perform in preparation for the competition of their lives. You too might have a ritual, a personal saying or mantra, or a special experience that you recall that lets you channel positive energy into your athletic experience. You may have a lucky pair of socks, a favorite song to listen to, or a mantra that charges you up. Find out whatever works for you and use it.

WRITE DOWN HERE WHAT WORKS FOR YOU.

_____

_____

_____

Develop pre-event rituals. Before your competition, do whatever makes you comfortable. Finding what specific pre-event routine works for you will require some trial and error, but key components include relaxation, visualization, and breathing exercises.

You may want to visualize the course or the race and see an image of yourself competing and doing well. Mutola listens to recordings by reggae artist Bob Marley to focus while rehearsing her race, her breathing, and her positive energy. She knows that she is ready to race and that "everything's gonna be all right" when all of these pieces come together. Evans uses breathing and relaxation techniques at the start of races to help herself get ready to race. Cyclist Karl Maxon factors visualization and proper breathing techniques into specific and deeply focused imagery practice before he races.

WORKSHEET: MENTAL TRAINING
FOR YOUR SPORT

Use this worksheet to apply mental practice to sports not covered in this book.

Use affirmations and self-talk. Practice these during training as well as competition. Tell yourself, "I can do this." Don't allow negative thoughts. Choose a cue word or phrase such as "You can do it" to use during tough times.

WRITE DOWN HERE WHAT WORKS FOR YOU.

_____

_____

_____

Breathe right. Practice full breathing regularly (see Chapter 4 for specific practice steps). Before your event, you may want to listen to a specific piece of music to practice relaxed, comfortable breathing. You might pair an image, such as crossing the finish line of a race or seeing yourself climbing powerfully, with your breathing routine.

WRITE DOWN HERE WHAT WORKS FOR YOU.

_____

_____

_____

Meditate. Meditation during a race or training will help you shut out the outside world and concentrate on your own event. Choose a mantra to repeat before and during the race to help you concentrate and stay relaxed.

WRITE DOWN HERE WHAT WORKS FOR YOU.

_____

_____

_____

Relax. After hard workouts, practice progressive relaxation to relax your muscles. Establish your own relaxation routine with an audiotape. Practice a mini relaxation session, perhaps using deep breaths or counting backward from 10 to calm yourself or relax a tense muscle. Practice relaxing during training so you can call up the relaxation response to calm yourself, if needed, during competition.

WRITE DOWN HERE WHAT WORKS FOR YOU.

_____

_____

_____

Practice imagery and visualization. To begin guided imagery, identify how you view images by filling out the questionnaire on page 56. For imagery practice, videotape yourself or tape your sport when it's shown on television.

WRITE DOWN HERE WHAT WORKS FOR YOU.

_____

_____

_____

Consider your opponents. Mentally visualize the person or people you'll be competing against. Study their strengths and weaknesses. See yourself performing strongly against that person or team.

WRITE DOWN HERE WHAT WORKS FOR YOU.

_____

_____

_____

Visualize technique. During your mental training sessions, carefully watch yourself perform each step of your sport. If you know you have a particular weakness, mentally practice doing that part of your sport flawlessly.

WRITE DOWN HERE WHAT WORKS FOR YOU.

_____

_____

_____

Build a victory image. Imagine what it will feel like to win your event or defeat a tough competitor. Experience the sight, sound, and feel of that winning experience.

WRITE DOWN HERE WHAT WORKS FOR YOU.

_____

_____

_____

Use visual motor behavior rehearsal (VMBR). Visualize yourself in a competition; focus on enhancing your technique and analyzing and mentally correcting errors. While training, practice the corrected behavior. Before events, imagine all the details of the competition and how you will meet challenges that might arise. Practice switching back and forth between a relaxed phase and a ready-to-win state of mind (see page 65 for specific steps).

WRITE DOWN HERE WHAT WORKS FOR YOU.

_____

_____

_____

Have a pre-event routine. Anticipate, prepare for, and minimize as many distractions as possible. At the competition site, check out the surroundings, the crowd, the weather, and the noise. Look around to see who your competitors are. Thirty minutes before the start, move into your PTEZ, or perfect timing and energy zone. Block out the past and the future and focus on the present. Practice relaxed breathing; visualize yourself competing and doing well. Tell yourself that you will compete as well as you ever have before. Do any pre-event rituals that make you more comfortable.

WRITE DOWN HERE WHAT WORKS FOR YOU.

_____

_____

_____

GUIDED IMAGERY FOR ANY SPORT

Before using any mental practice strategy, it's important to get very comfortable and relaxed. Sit in your favorite easy chair, and be sure that you will not be distracted for 30 to 45 minutes. This is your alone time.

Begin by breathing deeply and without strain. Imagine yourself at the site where you will be competing. Regardless of the site—across town or across the ocean—create a strong mental image of the environment. Imagine yourself wearing your favorite warmup gear, including your favorite hat or any good-luck piece of clothing that you enjoy wearing.

Then, while breathing comfortably, notice the conditions of the competition site: the heat or coolness, the atmosphere, and the humidity. Get a good reading on your own internal and external thermometer. Then begin to picture the other competitors in your event. As you begin to notice these athletes, tune in to the way you feel and allow yourself to get completely comfortable, confident, and ready to take on the world. Notice the calm that comes into your mind when you see the other competitors in your preparatory images.

Next, still sitting quietly in your armchair, move your imagery to your stretches and warmup place. Notice how relaxed you feel when you begin to stretch your arms and legs and prepare for the big event. Feel the confidence filter onto your imagery screen as you allow all the tension to leave your extremities. As you complete your warmups, move to the start of your event. In your mind's eye, take a good look at all the competitors, see their faces and expressions, and notice their eyes. You may feel some excitement at this point, so continue to enjoy this excitement and surge of energy; it is natural and very much a part of your preparation.

As you see your competitors getting ready to compete, notice how comfortable and supremely confident you feel. You are ready to compete, and you are not burdened with anxiety. You possess just the right amount of competitive energy. Next, take your images to the actual event and the heat of the competition. Notice how you feel when you get into position after your event gets underway. Check out your body and the fluid motion of your arms and legs, and be certain to make contact with the athletes you need to keep an eye on. Take your clear and comfortable images through your entire event. See yourself playing a perfect game or doing a perfect race, in perfect form, and winning with grace and ease. Notice the ease of your breathing, the lightness of your feet, and the agility of your limbs. Allow yourself to soak up the pleasure and delight of winning this competition. See, hear, and feel the crowd, using all of your sensory input; and enjoy their appreciation of you and your accomplishment.

Congratulations! You have just won the event of your life! Gradually and slowly end your imagery session with several deep and comfortable breaths. Experience the renewed confidence you feel as you reenter the room and the space around you. Enjoy this feeling. Now it's time to get ready for your training workout.

Elite athletes usually perform this 30- to 45-minute exercise every day. Recreational athletes report doing some form of mental preparation on the day of their races. Whatever your schedule or rhythm for mental preparation and imagery rehearsal, know that it works and believe in the strategy. It is fun, relaxing, and a great way to prepare for workouts.

RESOURCES

Guided imagery should be part of your regular physical training regimen and is best initiated under the supervision of a qualified coach or facilitator. To set up a guided imagery program, you can ask a licensed professional to assist you or your team. To help you locate coaches or facilitators for your particular sport, contact the parent organization or federation for your sport from the list below.

ARCHERY:

USA Archery (National Archery Association)
One Olympic Plaza
Colorado Springs, CO 80909
Phone: 719-866-4576
Fax: 719-632-4733
www.usarchery.org
Executive director: Bradley R. Camp
Phone: 719-866-4577
BCamp@usarchery.org

BADMINTON:

USA Badminton
One Olympic Plaza
Colorado Springs, CO 80909
Phone: 719-866-4808
Fax: 719-866-4507
www.usabadminton.org
Executive director: Dan Cloppas
Phone: 719-866-4808 Ext. 2
DCloppas@aol.com

BASEBALL:

USA Baseball
PO Box 1131
Durham, NC 27702
Phone: 919-474-8721
Fax: 919-474-8822
www.usabaseball.com
Executive director: Paul V. Seiler
PaulSeiler@usabaseball.com

BASKETBALL:

USA Basketball
5465 Mark Dabling Boulevard
Colorado Springs, CO 80918-3842
Phone: 719-590-4800
Fax: 719-590-4811
www.usabasketball.com
Executive director: Jim Tooley

BIATHLON:

US Biathlon Association
29 Ethan Allen Avenue
Colchester, VT 05446
Phone: 802-654-7833
Fax: 802-654-7830
www.usbiathlon.org
Consultant: Stephen Sands
Phone: 802-654-7833
USBiathlon@aol.com

BOXING:

USA Boxing
One Olympic Plaza
Colorado Springs, CO 80909
Phone: 719-866-4506
Fax: 719-632-3426
www.usaboxing.org

CANOE AND KAYAK:

USA Canoe/Kayak
301 South Tryon Street
Suite 1750
Charlotte, NC 28282
Phone: 704-348-4330
Fax: 704-348-4418
www.usack.org
Executive director: David
Yarborough
Dmyarborough@usack.org

CYCLING:

USA Cycling
One Olympic Plaza
Colorado Springs, CO 80909
Phone: 719-866-4581
Fax: 719-866-4628 or 719-866-
4596
www.usacycling.org
Chief executive officer:
Gerard Bisceglia
GBisceglia@usacycling.org

DIVING:

United States Diving, Inc.
201 South Capitol Avenue, Suite 430
Indianapolis, IN 46225
Phone: 317-237-5252
Fax: 317-237-5257
www.usadiving.org
Executive director: Todd Smith
Todd.Smith@usadiving.org

FENCING:

United States Fencing Association
One Olympic Plaza
Colorado Springs, CO 80909-5774
Phone: 719-866-4511
Fax: 719-632-5737
www.usfencing.org
Executive director: Michael Massik
Michael.Massik@USFencing.org

FIELD HOCKEY:

US Field Hockey Association
One Olympic Plaza
Colorado Springs, CO 80909
Phone: 719-866-4567
Fax: 719-632-0979
www.usfieldhockey.com
Executive director: Sheila Walker
SWalker@usfieldhockey.com

FIGURE SKATING:

United States Figure Skating
Association (USFSA)
20 First Street
Colorado Springs, CO 80906
Phone: 719-635-5200
Fax: 719-635-9548
www.usfsa.org

GYMNASTICS:

USA Gymnastics
Pan American Plaza, Suite 300
201 South Capitol Avenue
Indianapolis, IN 46225
Phone: 317-237-5050
Fax: 317-237-5069
www.usa-gymnastics.org

HOCKEY:

USA Hockey, Inc.
1775 Bob Johnson Drive
Colorado Springs, CO 80906-4090
Phone: 719-576-USAH (8724)
Fax: 719-538-1160
www.usahockey.com

JUDO:

USA Judo National Office
One Olympic Plaza, Suite 202
Colorado Springs, CO 80909
Phone: 719-866-4730
Fax 719-866-4733
www.usjudo.org
President: Dr. Ron Tripp
DrRonTripp@aol.com

KARATE:

USA Karate Federation
1300 Kenmore Boulevard
Akron, OH 44314
Phone: 330-753-3114
Fax: 330-753-6967
www.usakarate.org

ORIENTEERING:

US Orienteering Federation
PO Box 1444
Forest Park, GA 30298
Phone: 404-363-2110
www.us.orienteering.org
President: Chuck Ferguson
Fergusoncm@tecom.usmc.mil

PENTATHLON:

Pentathlon USA
5415 Bandera Road, Suite 512
San Antonio, Texas 78238
Phone: 210-229-2004
Fax: 210-647-7194
www.usapentathlon.org
Executive director: Robert Marbut
Assistant: Charlene Loeffler

RACQUETBALL:

US Racquetball Association
1685 West Uintah
Colorado Springs, CO 80904-2906
Phone: 719-635-5396
Fax: 719-635-0685
www.racquetball.org
Executive director: Jim Hiser
JHiser@usra.org

ROWING:

US Rowing
201 South Capitol Avenue
Suite 400
Indianapolis, IN 46225
Phone: 800-314-4769
Fax: 317-237-5646
www.usrowing.org

SAILING:

United States Sailing Association
PO Box 1260
15 Maritime Drive
Portsmouth, RI 02871-0907
Phone: 401-683-0800
www.ussailing.org
Executive director: Charlie
Leighton
CLeighton@ussailing.org

SKIING:

US Ski and Snowboard Association
Box 100
1500 Kearns Boulevard
Park City, UT 84060
Phone: 435-649-9090
Fax: 435-649-3613
www.ussa.org
President/chief executive officer:
Bill Marolt
BMarolt@ussa.org

SOCCER:

US Soccer Federation
1801 South Prairie Avenue
Chicago, IL 60616
Phone: 312-808-1300
Fax: 312-808-1301
www.ussoccer.org
Executive director: Dan Flynn
DFlynn@ussoccer.org

SOFTBALL:

Amateur Softball Association
2801 Northeast 50th Street
Oklahoma City, OK 73111
Phone: 405-425-3431
Fax: 405-424-4734
www.asasoftball.com
Executive director: Ron Radigonda
RRadigonda@softball.org

SPEED SKATING:

US Speedskating
PO Box 450639
Westlake, OH 44145
Phone: 440-899-0128
Fax: 440-899-0109
www.usspeedskating.org
Executive director: Katie Marquard
KMarquard@usspeedskating.org

SWIMMING:

USA Swimming
One Olympic Plaza
Colorado Springs, CO 80909
Phone: 719-866-4578
Fax: 719-866-4669
www.usaswimming.org
Executive director: Chuck Wielgus
CWielgus@usa-swimming.org

TABLE TENNIS:

United States Table Tennis
Association (USTTA)
One Olympic Plaza
Colorado Springs, CO 80909
Phone: 719-866-4583
Fax: 719-632-6071
www.usatt.org
Executive director: Doru Gheorghe
ed@usatt.org

TAE KWON DO:

United States Taekwondo Union
(USTU)
1 Olympic Plaza
Suite 104C
Colorado Springs, CO 80909
Phone: 719-866-4632
Fax: 719-866-4642
www.ustu.org

TENNIS:

United States Tennis Association
70 West Red Oak Lane
White Plains, NY 10604
Phone: 914-696-7000
www.usta.com
Executive director and chief
operating officer: Lee Hamilton
Hamilton@usta.com

TRACK AND FIELD:

USA Track and Field
One RCA Dome, Suite 140
Indianapolis, IN 46225
Phone: 317-261-0500
Fax: 317-261-0514
www.usatf.org
Chief executive officer: Craig
Masback
Craig.Masback@usatf.org

TRIATHLON:

USA Triathlon National Office
1365 Garden of the Gods Road
Suite 250
Colorado Springs, CO 80907
Phone: 719-597-9090
Fax: 719-597-2121
www.usatriathlon.org

VOLLEYBALL:

United States Volleyball Association
(USVBA)
715 South Circle Drive
Colorado Springs, CO 80910-1740
Phone: 719-228-6800
Fax: 719-228-6899
www.usavolleyball.org
President: Albert M. Monaco, Jr.
Al.Monaco@usav.org

WATER SKIING:

American Water Ski Association
(AWSA)
1251 Holy Cow Road
Polk City, FL 33868
Phone: 863-324-4341
Fax: 863-325-8259
www.usawaterski.org
Executive director: Steve McDermeit
SMcDermeit@usawaterski.org

WEIGHT LIFTING:

USA Weightlifting, Inc.
One Olympic Plaza
Colorado Springs, CO 80909
Phone: 719-866-4508
Fax: 719-866-4741
www.usaweightlifting.org
Executive director: Wesley Barnett
WesBarnett@usaweightlifting.org

WRESTLING:

USA Wrestling (USAW)
6155 Lehman Drive
Colorado Springs, CO 80918
Phone: 719-598-8181
Fax: 719-598-9440
www.usawrestling.org
Executive director: Rich Bender
RBender@usawrestling.org

FOR DRUG INFORMATION AND THE USE OF NUTRITIONAL SUPPLEMENTS AND VITAMINS

United States Anti-Doping Agency
(USADA)
Phone: 800-233-0393
www.usantidoping.org

World Anti-Doping Agency
(WADA)
Phone: 514-904-9232
www.wada-ama.org
code@wada-ama.org

Call your local family doctor and/or
sports medicine physician.

INDEX

Underscored page references indicate boxed text.

AUTHOR BIOGRAPHY

Steven Ungerleider, PhD, author of six books, completed his undergraduate studies in psychology at the University of Texas, Austin, where he also competed as a collegiate gymnast. He holds master's and doctorate degrees from the University of Oregon and is a licensed psychologist at Integrated Research Services in Eugene, Oregon.

Since 1984, he has served on the United States Olympic Committee Sport Psychology Registry and was recently appointed to the World Anti-Doping Agency's Education and Ethics Committee.

Ungerleiders' books include: *Beyond Strength* (McGraw-Hill, 1991, with coauthor Jacqueline Golding, PhD) and *Quest for Sucess* (WRS/Spence Publications, 1994). *Mental Training for Peak Performance*, First Edition, his third book (Rodale Press, 1996), was named to the book of the month club selection for *Men's Health* magazine.

In the early 1990s, Ungerleider was invited to join an international team of researchers to examine the East German doping files, monitor the criminal trials, and interview hundreds of witnesses for his fourth book entitled *Faust's Gold: Inside the East German Doping Machine* (St. Martin's Press).

In December 2001, *Faust's Gold* was honored as top "sports book of the year" by *Runner's World*. Ungerleider's work has been reviewed in *Elle, Longevity, Outside, Runner's World, Allure, New York Daily News, San Francisco Chronicle, Boston Herald, Dallas Morning News, New York Times, Chicago Tribune, Los Angeles Times, New Yorker* magazine, *Sports Illustrated, International Herald Tribune, People* magazine, *Forbes* magazine, *Washington Post, Newsweek*, and National Public Radio.

Ungerleider's East German doping research is the subject of a one-hour documentary by the Canadian Film Company, as well as a one-hour special by ABC's *20/20*, and NOS of Dutch Television.

Ungerleider can be reached at: suinteg@attglobal.net.